Food Additives

Food Additives

R.J. Taylor
Formerly of Unilever Research

JOHN WILEY & SONS
Chichester · New York · Brisbane · Toronto

British Library Cataloguing in Publication Data:
Taylor, Reginald James
    Food additives.—(The Institution of
    Environmental Sciences. Series).
    1. Food additives
    I. Title   II. Series
    664'.06   TX553.A3   79–42729

    ISBN 0 471 27684 7 (Cloth)
    ISBN 0 471 27683 9 (Paper)

Typeset by Preface Ltd, Salisbury, Wilts.
and printed in the United States of America

Introduction to Series

In the last two decades the environment has figured increasingly in our everyday discussions. From a matter of superficial interest to all but an enlightened few, it has become not just the calling of professors and politicians, but the concern of parliaments and the responsibility of us all. This explosive increase of interest has been associated with an ever-widening accumulation of related environmental facts. This series seeks to bring together these facts, and allied ideas, so that they may be readily accessible in a number of identifiable volumes. The Institution of Environmental Sciences in promoting the series has, as an objective, the express desire to diffuse a balanced professional view on all matters relating to the environment.

The environment now figures prominently as a curriculum subject and Environmental Science is established as a school and university examination subject at all levels. The need for a comprehensive series of volumes which disseminate the wealth of information relating to this science has become of paramount importance. The series should be of value both to students of the environment and to professionals working in related fields.

PETER FARAGO
DAVID HUGHES-EVANS
JOHN F. POTTER

Preface

This text has been prepared to provide an objective assessment of current practice in the use of food additives. Its intention is both to inform interested laypeople and to instruct science students. It has been written within the context of world food supplies and their historical development, of legal controls and of safety testing, and in this it differs from all other treatments of food additives known to the author. Obviously some knowledge of chemistry and of the underlying chemical basis of nutrition will be an advantage to the reader, but the concepts involved have been presented as simply as possible to widen its appeal, albeit without loss of scientific authority. It is not a handbook on the use of additives for those active in the food industry. Likewise, it is not a handbook on current legislation on food additives, for which the appropriate regulations should always be consulted. Its purpose is to provide readers with an overall picture of food additives that will lead to an understanding of their *raison d'être* and of the controls that condition the use of them.

Contents

Introduction

Why should the subject of food additives be classed as an environmental science? This may puzzle some readers as much as it has provided food for thought for the author. On consideration I see that there is a case to be made. The environment is something that calls for value judgements as well as scientific understanding. And value judgements are conditioned as much by personal susceptibilities and emotive response as by objective reasoning. So discussions about the environment are very much battles for the mind: to confirm it in, or wean it from, its susceptibilities.

In a similar way, food additives invoke value judgements, and indeed there has been a surfeit of them in popular and pseudo-scientific writings. But what of truly scientific understanding? And who am I to be contributing to it? Peering back through the mists of time I recall that once, long ago, I attended a meeting that the then Ministry of Food had called to discuss food colours. Professor R. A. Morton was also there, and I realize in retrospect that I was present at the conception, if not the birth, of the U.K. Food Additives and Contaminants Committee, of which Professor Morton became chairman. And when I look at the list of substances now called additives—vitamins, colours, flavours, preservatives, antioxidants, and so on—I realize that I have been very actively involved with a number of them on and off during much of my research life, but I never thought of them as additives, but rather as substances adding to the quality of food, and it pleased me that we were engaged in that kind of work. I have to confess that, in my naivety, and as part of my philosophy, I thought at first that substances extracted from a natural food source, and synthetic copies of them, were safe for addition to another food. And it surprised me that such rigorous testing should be needed before synthetic vitamin A should be approved. I had become indoctrinated by the time we identified δ-lactones as natural food flavours, and confirmed in my indoctrination when we found that certain other constituents of a very popular food product were inadmissable as additives elsewhere.

Expositions on additives exist. Indeed if they did not this book could not have been written, for my own experience could not possibly span the whole range of them. But the information is scattered, and appears in books and journals not readily available. Furthermore, most of it is written for experts, often in terms that only they understand. There is a need for a book therefore at a more popular level, which provides balanced scientific assessment of the need for additives, and puts them into context with human needs over the centuries, particularly in conserving and using to the best advantage his sources of food. This has been my guiding principle while writing the text.

Admittedly, the situation has not been helped by man's own occasional roguery that has led him at times to contaminate food for the sake of profit. But this has been stamped out to all intents and purposes within what we are pleased to call the civilized world, and laws and public conscience keep a tight hold. However, it is still active in developing countries, and presents a complicating factor, particularly as those who dislike additives look on them as contaminants. It is important therefore that an additive should be clearly recognized for what it is: something put into food to protect or enhance its value, or to make it more attractive as a food.

Inevitably the question of safety arises, but that does not concern only additives. It applies to all our food supplies: The World Health Organization has rightly observed:

'It is generally recognized that all chemicals (which include foods) are toxic to animals and man if large enough doses are administered. Even so-called innocous substances when given in excessive doses, may induce specific untoward effects as a result of various unspecific actions, e.g. physical obstruction of the gastrointestinal tract, alteration of osmotic pressure, and nutritional imbalance. A limit in the daily intake of a substance is essential for the health of the consumer.'

So a check is needed, but really no more so for additives than for common sources of food. Yet people consume such sources quite happily, oblivious of the occasional risk to which they may be exposed. It is only additives that have come under public scrutiny and criticism, and this has led to an ever-increasing regimen of safety testing with the passing of time. Not that all tests will give clear-cut answers. Life is not like that. Not everyone catches flu, or measles, or mumps, when the viruses make their annual round, even though exposure is uniform. We live on a probability basis, and the higher the probability of a hazard, the more necessary it becomes to take action. So with additives: the higher the risk, the more certain it is that they should not be permitted: the lower the risk, the easier it is to lay down conditions for safe use.

There is general agreement throughout the world on the aims to be achieved by controlling the use of additives, but there are varying ideas on what should be controlled and how it should be done. This is not immediately obvious, for the literature on the subject is voluminous, and only when salient facts are isolated do gaps appear in the structural pattern. This has made it difficult therefore to present as coherent a picture of the world situation as one would have wished, or as critical a comparison of procedures as one would have liked. Nevertheless, the picture that does emerge should leave no one in doubt that it is getting as hard for a suspect additive to get through the safety net as it ever was for the proverbial camel to squeeze through the eye of a needle.

In dealing with the subject at the chosen level of exposition, namely, for students entering college or university, it has been taken to be a prime necessity to get additives into proper perspective as part of the total problem throughout recorded history—and earlier through archaeological evidence—of improving and maximizing food supplies. In order to do this it is necessary to say something of the origins and development of organized food resources, for it is unlikely that many readers' earlier studies will have acquainted them with this. A concise treatment had therefore been given which enables a comparison to be made between the attitudes towards food and towards additives.

Insofar as those additives that are currently permitted are a consequence of legal enactments and safety testing, it would have been more logical to deal with these matters before coming to the additives themselves. But it has been thought that to do so would have meant delaying treatment of the principal subject matter unduly. So they follow the chapter on additives. However, the book has been so written that it need not be read in sequence. Like Thomas Gray's famous line—The ploughman homeward plods his weary way—much may be transported without losing significance.

A word must be said here about what additives are defined to be, for this seems to have presented considerable difficulty to authorities, particularly when trying to put the definition into a legal framework. The reader will find three, or maybe four, different definitions in the text. For the purposes of this book additives are substances added purposely to food to preserve or enhance the value of the food, or to make it more palatable, and without detriment to its safety. They do not include pesticide residues or packaging plasticizers, etc. which are more properly contaminants and certainly not added purposely. Nevertheless, they are unlikely to escape the safety testing net described here if they should present a hazard.

The text is illustrated abundantly with formulae: partly because many of them would be difficult for readers to trace: partly because names without formulae are rather like faceless people: and partly because it is useful to observe that there are stranger substances occurring naturally in food than were ever put into it.

I wish to express my deep sense of gratitude to Dr. Ray Wilson and Miss Audrey Norris of Unilever Research for their advice, comment, and practical help in organizing source material, while dissociating them from the views expressed,. with which they may or may not agree. The plan and scope of the book are also mine, but the shaping of it owes much to them. Mrs Patsy Taylor also helped with the source material. I must also thank Unilever Research for permission to have these contacts with former colleagues. I have also to acknowledge helpful discussion, information, and comment from Dr. J. D. McGuinness, Dr. J. F. Howlett, and Dr. D. H. Buss of the Ministry of Agriculture, Fisheries and Food, and Dr. Sylvia J. Darke of the Department of Health and Social Security.

Finally I must thank the publishers for helping me to discover how much I had been involved with additives during my research activities.

R. J. TAYLOR

Obituary

Sadly, we mourn the passing of our former colleague Reg Taylor, and regret he was denied the opportunity to complete the publication of this book on food additives. We hope it will prove a fitting memorial of his many contributions to Science and Education.

R.W./J.A.N.

CHAPTER 1

The Origins and Development of Food Sources

It is generally considered, by those most competent to assess the evidence, that our remotest ancestors—or most of them—relied for subsistence solely on a variety of wild fruits, seeds, nuts, roots, insects, honey, and on such wild animals as could be caught by hand. They may have been able to avoid some poisonous plants by observing what happened to animals that ate them but, insofar as casual animal response is not a certain guide to human safety, it is very likely that some people acted unwittingly as guinea pigs in the struggle for survival. It is very likely too that the survivors would come to recognize not only those plants that would kill them—and the more unscrupulous among them to use them for the acquisition of power—but also those that would make them ill. What they could not do—nor indeed could modern man till quite recently—was to recognize delayed toxic effects of specific, seemingly edible, plants when eaten to excess or as a staple source of food. It cannot be said yet that all have now been recognized.

It is likely that winters took a hard toll on such diets. A favoured few, according to archaeological evidence,[1] had learnt to make tools and kill larger animals at least two million years ago. But animal meat in those days, and fish for those to whom it was available, must have been eaten raw, for evidence of hearth fires does not date back more than 56,000 years, and that evidence suggests that such fires were used more to keep warm and scare off wild animals than to cook food. Indeed we have to come to a period of no more than 20,000 years ago before evidence emerges that man was in control of fire and using it systematically to cook. It coincides with the appearance of so-called Cro-Magnon man, a sort of 'mark 1' modern man, with a brain power capable of exploiting his environment with some intelligence. Unfortunately he was not able to do so to any great extent because his world was still passing through the Ice Age. In the interim—a very long interim of 10,000 years—he hunted intensively, with fire helping to make his food more digestible and palatable.

Fortunately the Ice Age did come to an end for, as Bernal has pointed

1

out,[2] 'The essential weakness of a hunting society is that it is parasitic on the animals it hunts. It can kill off the animals, but it cannot feed them or make them breed.' We have a similar situation approaching today with whales, and we are in incipient danger of one with fish.

With the ending of the Ice Age man was able at long last to develop the arts of agriculture, albeit at first in a very primitive way, but he did devise ways of making a number of hitherto toxic plants edible, and all plants more digestible and, with the domestication of animals that followed, the danger of overhunting receded. It is implicit in this that the 'fruits' of the earth were originally works of nature in their own right, with their own survival, defence, and reproductive mechanisms. Early man, for his own continued survival, found by a crude system of cause and effect what was good for him to eat, what could be made good, and what was to be avoided.

It was about 10,000 years ago that he began organizing his food resources, observing the conditions under which seed sprouted in the spring, and noting that selected seed yielded increasingly better quality and quantity. This presupposes sources of wild seed and, for cereals, it has been argued that the likeliest sources were those where the greatest varieties of wild plants still grow today. It is worth noting in passing that there is a resurgence of interest in the primitive forebears not only of cereals but of all vegetable crops,[3] for the plant breeding revolution that has led to high-yielding modern crops has resulted also in the loss of such useful characteristics as disease resistance. So the search is on for sources of primitive species from which to create a genetic bank of desirable characteristics which plant breeders can make use of in their future work.

So far as wheat is concerned it seems that the soft varieties originated in the mountain valleys of Persia and Afghanistan, and hard varieties in Ethiopia. Migrants brought supplies of both types of grain down to Egypt and Mesopotamia, and subsequent migration waves took them into Europe: first westward along the Mediterranean, then northward towards Scandinavia. The sources were contaminated with oats, barley, and rye; hardier plants that did better than wheat in the more northerly lands.

The contaminant cereals were not popular in warmer climates, particularly oats which, having a higher fat content, tended to go rancid. Seemingly, however, even in those far-off days, there were embryonic food processors about, with an eye for a good food additive, for there is evidence of liquor made from malted grains in Mesopotamia around 8000 years ago. And there are Egyptian records of 5000 years ago describing the brewing of beer from barley. This must be the first recorded use of an additive, yeast. And that was soon to be followed by other additives for it was an early practice to put in flavour principles, as hops are put in today. The Egyptians also found that they could make leavened bread with yeast, thus putting the same additive to different uses. It is likely that salt came into use as an additive to food about this time, as a seasoning rather than something supplying a physiological need. Egyptian brewers doubled up as bakers—or *vice versa.* Today the trades are well separated, and even the yeast for the one product would not do for the other.

Cultivation first began in river silt systems and then spread to terraced hills in the belief that only water was required and irrigation could replace the natural river flow. Many centuries were to pass before it was discovered why the terraces became infertile and had to be replaced periodically, while river cultivation continued to flourish. The introduction of manuring changed all that, but more centuries had to pass before it became known what manuring did and artificial fertilizers could be made.

In the interim another kind of progress was made, in the development of other food sources: rice and various millets in the Far East, and maize in Central America. An instinctive need for fats was met in temperate zones by animal fats, including mild fat, and in warmer climates by see oils such as those of the poppy, sesame, olive, almond, peach, and apricot. The vine, cabbage, beetroot, turnip, radish, onion, and garlic came into cultivation about 4000 years ago, and so did the legumes, peas and lentils. The first cultivation of groundnuts, native to Brazil, is not known, but the now rival soya bean appeared in Chinese records over 4,500 years ago.

In the soya bean we have a classic example of the use of fire to cook and make edible an otherwise toxic plant, for the Chinese quickly learnt to make what for them were attractive and safe food dishes, including a soya milk. Furthermore they discovered how to prevent scurvy by allowing beans to shoot, for the young shoots contained vitamin C. Not that people in more northerly coniferous zones were far behind in this for they discovered that an infusion of fresh pine needles was equally beneficial. Wild edible fruit and vegetables also made a contribution.

We see then that by the dawn of history, in centres of emergent civilization, man was gaining some control over his environment, to the extent that he had a range of foods available to him that went a considerable way towards providing him—albeit unknowingly—with a reasonably satisfactory diet in nutritional terms. And though, in succeeding centuries, he vastly improved his systems of agriculture and animal management (not everywhere, of course, for very primitive systems are still followed in parts of the world today), and migrations and conquests spread this knowledge around, he marked time nutritionally. This is not really surprising when we bring to mind the relatively brutal times in which he lived. Death from inadequate nutrition would be no more than one of a number of likely causes of premature decease—war, violence, premeditated poisoning, disease—and life expectation was quite short. Furthermore the handling of food, and culinary expertise, were not of a high order, and we find herbs and spices, prized primarily for their medicinal qualities, being used to disguise the taints and off-flavours of foods. Another era of food additives had begun.

So had the age of organized roguery as society became more dependent on a food trade. One can deduce that there have been rogues from the earliest times for there is evidence in ancient Chinese, Hindu, Greek, and Roman writings of attempts to prevent adulteration and fraudulent description.[4] Beer and wine were prime targets for dishonest merchants; and bread, fish, and milk did not escape their attentions either. In all this the authorities were concerned not only to prevent fraud but also to ensure, as best they could, that unwholesome food of any kind did not reach the consumer. The Mosaic rules on the matter enshrined in biblical history are evidence of this.

Not that there was any once-for-all victory for there was always someone set to exploit loopholes in the rules. The establishment of Trade Guilds in Britain in the Middle Ages had for its purpose to set standards of competence and integrity, and butchers, bakers, brewers, cooks, and retailers of fruit and vegetables became guild members sworn to maintain standards. So the skirmishing proceeded throughout the ensuing centuries between those who thought the adulteration of food to be no more than a matter of commercial astuteness and those who saw it as a hazard to health. Not till modern times did it cease to be a problem in developed countries, though alas it still remains so elsewhere, but it is interesting to reflect that present-day food and food additive laws and regulations are in a direct line of descent from the earliest attempts to ensure wholesome sources of food.

Such attempts were necessarily limited in their understanding of what was needed for it was not until the 19th century that any knowledge of the nutritional purpose of food began to emerge. Scheele and Lavoisier had laid the foundations of biochemistry at the end of the 18th century, and Liebig, in the early part of the 19th century, established the relevance of carbon chemistry to it. The three main components of living matter, and hence of food—proteins, carbohydrates, and fats—had been identified by the time Emil Fischer appeared on the scene, but it was he who both directed and participated in the work that led to the recognition that proteins were compounds of amino acids, carbohydrates of simple sugars, and fats of fatty acids. When the biological significance of all this was recognized it became possible to attach nutritional meaning to the various categories of food that people ate: meat, vegetables, cereals, and so on.

The simple ideas that emerged, however, were rudely shaken at the beginning of the 20th century when Gowland Hopkins put forward his ideas on accessory food factors to explain the cure for scurvy and the prevention of rickets. One by one the vitamins were discovered and named, and related to the deficiency disease that each led to *in absentia*. This led to a recognition that many diets could be missing in essential nutrients and yet another era in food additives was ushered in.

Let us exemplify this with margarine which was devised originally just prior to the Franco-Prussian war to make up for critical shortages of butter. We know now that butter is a useful source of vitamins A and D, and of the provitamin β-carotene (though how much depends on whether it is a summer or winter butter). But it was not known then and margarine was made as a simple emulsion of fat, water, salt, and skimmed milk, together with a little minced cow's stomach. Composition and method of manufacture improved over the years, but the presence of vitamins in butter was not discovered till just prior to the 1914–18 war, and it was not until the 1920s that enlightened manufacturers—without government prompting—put them successfully into margarine. The addition became compulsory in the 1940s.

Next came the discovery that certain amino acids and fatty acids must be present in the diet if an optimum nutritional balance is to be maintained, since the body is not able to synthesize them from ingested food. The quality of proteins and fats was then seen to be as important as the quantity. Later still, it was found that certain trace elements were also essential, but how best to deal with these—in terms of additives—is still unclear. Not only is it fortuitous which elements an edible plant will contain, and how much of each, since it depends both on the geochemical character of the soil in which the plant was grown and the ability of the plant to assimilate one or other metal, but the borderline between essentiality and toxicity is narrow for some of them, e.g. selenium, and there are antagonisms and synergisms that affect the balance of power between those that are present. This does not diminish their importance, but it complicates their assessment.[5]

Nevertheless, from all this more recent knowledge has come a reasonably precise picture of optimum nutritional requirements, for groups ranging from infants and juveniles to adults in different conditions of living and working[6] (see Tables 1 and 2). It is up to agriculturalists and food processors to make available such a variety of food items as will allow nutritionists and dieticians to achieve their aims.

It is here that a word of caution must creep in. It has already been noted that plants were designed with their own survival in mind and not that of humans. This led Paracelsus, a famous physician and chemist of the 15th century, to remark—'All substances are poisons: there is none that is not a poison: the right dose differentiates a poison and a remedy': a remark that

Table 1. Protein Requirements: Minimum and Recommended Intakes. (Source: *Recommended Intakes of Nutrients for the United Kingdom*, H.M.S.O., London, 1969)

Age group	Minimum (g/day)		Recommended (g/day)	
	start	rising to	start	rising to
Birth/12 months	13	16	20	20
1/9 years	19	30	30	53
9/18 years (boys)	36	50	63	75
9/18 years (girls)	35	40	58	58
		Falling to		Falling to
18/75+ years (men)	45	38	68	53
18/75+ years (women)	38	34	55	48
Pregnancy	44		60	
Lactation	55		68	

Table 2. Minimum and Recommended Daily Intakes of Specific Vitamins and Minerals (based on U.S.F.D.A. regulation 21 CFR Parts 105.3, 105.85, Foods for Special Dietary Use (1977)—revoked March 16, 1979)

Nutrient	Dosage unit	Infants RDA	Children under 4 years min	Children under 4 years RDA	Adults + children 4 years or over min.	Adults + children 4 years or over RDA	Pregnancy + lactating women min.	Pregnancy + lactating women RDA
Vitamins—mandatory								
vitamin A	iu*	1500	1250	2500	2500	5000	5000	8000
vitamin D	iu	400	200	400			400	400
vitamin E	iu	5	5	10	15	30	30	30
vitamin C	mg	35	20	40	30	60	60	60
folic acid	mg	0.1	0.1	0.2	0.2	0.4	0.4	0.8
thiamine	mg	0.5	0.35	0.7	0.75	1.5	1.5	1.7
riboflavin	mg	0.6	0.4	0.8	0.8	1.7	1.7	2.0
niacin (nicotinic acid)	mg	8	4.5	9	10	20	20	20
vitamin B_6	mg	0.4	0.35	0.7	1	2	2	2.5
vitamin B_{12}	μg	2	1.5	3	3	6	6	8
Vitamins—optional								
vitamin D	iu				200	400		
biotin	mg	0.05	0.075	0.15	0.15	0.3	0.3	0.3
pantothenic acid	mg	3	2.5	5	5	10	10	10
Minerals—mandatory								
calcium	g	0.6	0.125	0.8	0.125	1	0.125	1.3
phosphorus	g	0.5	0.125	0.8	0.125	1		
iodine	μg	45	35	70	70	150	150	150
iron	mg	15	5	10	9	18	18	18
magnesium	mg	70	40	200	100	400	100	450
Minerals—optional								
phosphorus	g						0.125	1.3
copper	mg	0.6	0.5	1	1	2	1	2
zinc	mg	5	4	8	7.5	15	7.5	15

*iu = international unit.

has more than a grain of truth in it. And it has been said more recently—'It is clear that nothing is wholly safe or dangerous *per se*. It is the quantity involved, the manner and conditions of use, and the susceptibility of the organism which determine the degree of hazard or safety.[7] These people were not talking of food additives but of food itself.

The fact is that vitamins and the like are not the only minor constituents of food. Sources of food of all kinds contain small quantities of other naturally occurring chemicals, many of which are toxic to the human system. Some have been identified but there is much work to be done before it can be said for the whole range of foods what all those chemicals are and which are toxic. It is fortunate that the human system has become well adapted to a wide range of non-nutritional chemicals. It is well known, for example that it can build up quite a high tolerance to arsenic. It can inactivate, neutralize, or eliminate most chemical types, provided none is consumed in excessive amounts. However, when the commodity has become a major source of food, excess may well be consumed.

We are not considering here matters of acute toxicity, which even our remotest ancestors had learnt to recognize and avoid, but to those of chronic toxicity, of which it has been noted that 'long-delayed harmful effects of eating repeatedly certain natural foods remained a mystery until modern times. Relations between goitre, lathyrism, favism and ergotism and dietary food items were slow coming to light'[8] (see Appendix A). The same source has the following relevant comments also to make: 'If almost any of the specific non-nutritional chemicals found in food were to be tested in experimental animals by today's standards of safety, it would be shown to be toxic': and 'It is likely on a long-term basis that the margins of safety for natural toxins in our food are in many cases no greater, and in some cases considerably lower, than those legally permitted for food additives.' This is quoted, not to scare, but to get the matter of additives into perspective. In modern society we do not eat our food with any underlying feeling of hazard, nor should we have need of it.

Nevertheless, it is no defence of food additives to enumerate the potential hazards of ordinary food, or to point out that getting tanned in the sun, smoking, inhaling automobile fumes, or eating charcoal-cooked meats present more dangerous habits, or that the biggest killers are atherosclerosis, cancer, and obesity.[9] There has to be a positive case for the use of additives.

CHAPTER 2

The Case for Food Additives

Although, as Chapter 1 has shown, additives have been a feature of food preparation from very early times, the use of them has now grown into a very sophisticated science, and we need to examine the circumstances that led to this.

We live today in a world of widely different standards of affluence, and hence of differing attitudes towards food. There are communities that, through drought, flooding, famine or infertility of the soil, have insufficient and quite inadequate resources, and life for them is little more than existence at a starvation level. Others would have enough if they had the knowledge and aptitude to make the best of available resources, and life is not as satisfactory as it could be. Others again, smallish communities in Shangri La-like situations, live where the soil is fertile and can be kept so, the crops are good and the community is self-sufficient in food. Their diet could be improved with greater nutritional knowledge but they are reasonably well fed.

The remainder, the affluent society, as a consequence of the processes whereby it became affluent, has evolved to a way of life wherein the majority is dependent on a minority of suppliers for its food requirements. Not that all members of that society are affluent but, insofar as they are part of it, they are dependent on the system. This holds also for those who have ideas at variance with the majority—on the importance of organically grown food, for example—or who find satisfaction in tilling their own little plot of earth; for the system is not so rigid that it cannot accommodate them. However, it has evolved to meet the needs of that great majority who earn their living in non-agricultural activities: who lack 'green fingers', who work in towns and cities and commute daily from urban conurbations, and whose numbers include an ever-increasing number of women who have their own jobs and careers. The chance of being as well fed as anyone is theirs, but only if they do not let the ease of obtaining food blinker them to the need to take advantage of the nutritional knowledge and expertise made available by the affluence they have helped to create.

It all started with the Industrial Revolution and the drawing in of increasing numbers of people from the countryside to the towns, the consequential growth in the size and number of towns, and hence of populations not able to produce their own food. At first it meant no more than a reorganization of food supplies to match the redistribution of workers, but with the population explosion that followed, and the increased wealth that was generated, the situation changed. On the one hand, the demand for food grew beyond the capabilities of the older and smaller countries to remain self-sufficient. On the other the increased wealth (in an overall sense, for there have always been pockets of poverty among the wealth) burgeoned the demand for a greater variety of food, and hence for importing non-indigenous kinds of food in greater quantities. With the development of the prairie lands of the U.S.A. and Canada as wheat-growing areas came the realization that it made good economic sense to maximize industrial output at home and import more food from those areas better able to produce it.

At least, it seemed to make good economic sense at the time, but views have been modified by the impact of war and of periodic economic depression. So home production, boosted by advanced agricultural practices (that themselves have created new contaminant hazards), has achieved revived importance. But it is now more selective, and with a better balance between home-produced and imported foods. In Europe the formation of the EEC has meant that there will be further adjustments as the food programmes of the individual countries become more closely integrated. In all this the U.S. stands in splendid isolation as the one major country able to supply the bulk of its own sophisticated needs and to be a major exporter as well. (The U.S.S.R. could well join it if it were to direct more of its undoubted intelligence and ingenuity to the matter of food supply.) It is a matter of interest therefore that the U.S. should be in the forefront of work involving food additives.

Indeed, it is an indicator of the size of the problem facing the food industry. From its combined resources it has to cater for mass markets that require food not only for domestic consumption—and that often in the form of convenience foods—but also for restaurant, café, canteen, and school meal trade that constitutes so large a part of modern eating habits. It must be always on the look out for ways of holding food costs down. The family baker, butcher, pastrycook, and greengrocer still survive, and will continue to do so, particularly in small market towns. The art of home cooking and baking will continue to flourish. But all this is minimal in comparison with overall food requirements, and here the food supermarkets compete strongly in meeting demand. For these, many kinds of food need to be transported and stored in bulk, seasonal foods made available out of season, and fruit to be supplied ripe at the time of sale and not of harvesting.

So the affluent society has largely shaped the food industry as we know it today—an industry that must meet the requirements of that society as efficiently and economically as possible. It must provide food that is appetising and nutritious that would easily deteriorate if precautions were not taken. In support of those requirements it has undertaken research, not only into nutritional requirements, but also into food processing techniques that will help it to meet the demand. And food additives have played an important role there. What has to be ensured is that each is playing a role and not partaking in gimmickry.

At the same time, recognition by the more fortunate nations of a responsibility towards those that have been less favoured has led them, among other things, to devise world food aid programmes based on the nutritional knowledge and food formulation expertise they have acquired.[10] But it is not necessarily sufficient that the food should be nutritionally sound. Those working in the field[11] have found that, contrary to a commonly held belief that if people are hungry enough they will eat anything, the food must be liked and acceptable to those to whom it is offered.

Acceptability, in fact, is a more important attribute of food than many might think, often with community overtones. A U.K. manufacturer who was bold enough to leave added colour out of three food lines found sales to drop by about 50%.[12] And how would a children's party react to those popular, harmless and non-nutritive appetisers, table jellies, if they were without colour or flavour?

So the case for additives is this. All food, by the nature of it, is perishable sooner or later, and man has been concerned throughout history to conserve his resources; and from quite early times he has sought to enhance the palatability of it. Furthermore, as his knowledge of nutritional needs has grown, he has aimed to meet them by diversification of food sources and modification of food items. Now, in order to meet current food requirements, supplies must be organized and, if necessary, processed in ways that make the most efficient and economic use of resources, and provide food items that can be made up into attractive, appetising, and nutritionally balanced meals.

Admittedly, there are people who will argue against this approach, and will avoid preserved or processed foods as far as possible. But they are not concerned or involved in global requirements of food. They form a minority and, as such, their wishes can be met. World food supplies could never be organized on such lines, nor could world aid programmes. For the majority, therefore, it is fortunate that the food industry has become experienced in the use of additives, and thereby made available a wider selection of foods—and hence reduced monotony in the character of meals—than would otherwise have been possible. It can be argued that, not only has there not been any noticeably untoward effect from the consumption of food additives in food, but rather that, during a period of expanding use, there has been a consistent improvement in the general health and life expectation of people. This is not to claim a cause and effect situation but merely to reinforce the argument that additives have enabled food to make maximum nutritional impact.

As we have seen, there have been good historical precedents for the use of additives to maintain or even improve the quality of food, though the earliest were not concerned with preservation. (For this they relied on a primitive sun-drying process still in use in parts of the world today. Preservation with salt or vinegar followed later.) In using yeast to make beer or bread from cereals those early entrepreneurs were happy, in the one case, to have converted grain of doubtful keeping quality into a nutritious and sustaining drink, and in the other to have produced an easily digested food from a relatively indigestible grain. They were not to know that they had done better than they intended by the incidental inclusion of vitamins from the yeast: unpremeditated additives as it were.

When they brought spices and herbs into culinary practice the people of the time may well have been hoping for a double advantage, for the primary purpose of both spices and herbs was medicinal. They were used to blanket malodours and off-flavours—thus offering some insight into the general quality of food in those days—but no doubt it was nice to think that even if blanketing was only partially effective some other good had been achieved. And no doubt today, when blanketing is no longer an issue for most of us, and spices and herbs act as flavourings in their own right, the same sense of double advantage persists. Indeed some Indian curries are concocted with medicinal advantages in mind.

Salt could well have been the first ever additive for it is vital to a normal functioning of the human system and losses must be made good. It is said that the salt balance in the blood provides a clue to the period in time when our progenitors left the sea for a life of greater promise on land. It is certain that, once fixed in this whimsical manner, the balance needs to be maintained if the system is to continue functioning normally. It is probable, therefore, that the use of salt as a seasoning arose from a basic need to make good operational losses from the system. (In the great land masses of Central Asia salt has always been an important commercial commodity.)

One curious historical example of an unconscious use of additives was the burning of paraffin by the Chinese in ancient times to ripen fruit, the actual ripening agents being the combustion products, ethylene and propylene, which have been rediscovered and used in more recent times.[13]

The list of additives grew haphazardly over the centuries, but there were no more than 50 in the list at the beginning of the present century. It is a mark of the pace of change in food habits since then that it is now approaching 4000 items, though it must be added that, taking the individual flavour components of herbs and spices into account, the earlier list would add up to many more than 50, just as flavour components make up the major part of the present list. Later on we will be considering the consequences of this in some detail. Here it will suffice to note concisely that the list includes antioxidants, mould inhibitors, bactericides, emulsifiers, humectants, sweeteners, sequestering agents, colours, flavours, enzymes, and micronutrients.

12

To illustrate how the use of additives has grown to meet modern needs let us consider that example of early inventiveness and still popular commodity, bread. In the beginning only two additives were required, yeast and salt, and these sufficed for centuries, though many people found bread a useful carrier for other things, such as currants. The flour was wholemeal. When hard wheats became available in the U.K. after the repeal of the Corn Laws in 1846, millers found that they could so grind it as to eliminate both bran and wheat germ, leaving a whiter flour consisting wholly of endosperm. It was referred to in the trade as 72% extraction flour, wholemeal being 100%. The public much preferred the bread made from it, but it was a retrograde step nutritionally because two important B vitamins, and biologically available iron, were removed in the process. Although the importance of vitamins began to emerge at the beginning of the present century, and in time the limitations of 72% extraction flour were recognized, it was not till 1945 that action was taken to ensure that the errant vitamins—and the iron—were returned to the white bread, and the public remained contented.

At the same time, realizing how convenient a carrier bread was, it was decided that it should also be fortified with calcium, in the form of chalk, as a necessary minor dietary constituent to be available for bone formation.

More recently, other additives have been introduced to meet the needs of changing technology in breadmaking brought about by large-scale production, where the prime consideration is uniformity of raw materials and procedure. The wheats used are descendants of the hard and soft wheats of antiquity.

Only soft wheats grow well in the U.K. but hard wheats are preferred for breadmaking although, for economic reasons, it is best to use as much British wheat as possible. The hard wheats have a higher level of protein and it is this that gives bread its open elastic structure. So, to boost the protein, bakers add a small amount of soya flour (which contains a much higher level of protein) and this permits more British wheat to be used. At the same time it improves the level of three essential amino acids, lysine, leucine, and isoleucine.

Then there is the matter of aging, a mild oxidative process, formerly achieved by holding the flour for three or four weeks, but clearly inconvenient to large-scale working. The same effect is now obtained by adding a permitted 'improver' in a high-speed mixing machine. It is therefore no longer called aging but ripening.[15]

Next there is a yeast food to be added, to accelerate the fermentation process, and finally a mould inhibitor to improve the keepability of the baked loaf.

So, in its way, large-scale baking today epitomizes the role of food additives. They have enabled a product that forms a substantial part of the nation's diet to be produced in bulk to a prescribed standard, and in a keepable form that is acceptable to most of the population.

CHAPTER 3

The Character of Additives

In this chapter detailed consideration is given to the various classes of additives, particularly to what they do and what character is needed in order to do it; and why a multiplicity of substances in each class is needed to meet manufacturing requirements. It will be seen that the multiplicity varies from class to class, so that for some, all the permitted substances may be considered. With others the list is so large that selected substances must be illustratively used to convey the sense of the matter. Compilations, which give more exhaustive details than are possible here, are described in an appendix.

This means that the chapter should in no way be used as a guide to this or that additive, and indeed that is not its purpose. More information would be required and this is to be found in the more detailed original sources. The occasional reference to ADI, the acceptable daily intake for an additive, is illustrative. It does not mean that only those substances so referred to have ADIs. The purpose of the chapter is solely to help the reader understand why each class of additive is needed and how it does its job. The classes are identified as follows:

Antioxidants	Acids, buffers, and bases
Preservatives	Humectants
Emulsifiers and stabilizers	Firming and crisping agents
Food colours	Sweeteners
Flavours	Enzymes
Sequestrants	Nutritive additives
Anticaking agents	Flour and bread additives

Some protect the nutrient quality of the product, some enhance it. Some control texture, and some make it more attractive. Each has a positive impact.

Antioxidants

Antioxidants are used to protect unsaturated constituents of foods: mainly fats, though other substances, such as vitamins, also need protection. Some

13

readers may know what an unsaturated compound is: an organic substance based on carbon in which two or three of the four valency bonds of carbon link adjacent carbon atoms. Thus we have:

Ethane
$$
\begin{array}{ccc}
\text{H} & & \text{H} \\
| & & | \\
\text{H}-\text{C} & - & \text{C}-\text{H} \\
| & & | \\
\text{H} & & \text{H}
\end{array}
$$
a saturated compound, i.e. with all carbons bonded to different atoms (alkanes).

Ethene
$$
\begin{array}{ccc}
\text{H} & & \text{H} \\
| & & | \\
\text{C} & = & \text{C} \\
| & & | \\
\text{H} & & \text{H}
\end{array}
$$
in which the carbons are double bonded (alkenes).

Ethyne $\text{H}-\text{C}\equiv\text{C}-\text{H}$ in which the carbons are triple bonded (alkynes).

Discussion will be limited to compounds containing double bonds. Sometimes the compound is stable. Benzene, which contains six carbons in a ring, and double bonds alternating with single bonds in the ring, is an example. But when the carbons link together to form a chain, i.e. $-\text{C}-\text{C}=\text{C}-\text{C}-$, the compound is much less stable. The degree of instability depends on both the number of double bonds in the organic molecule and their positions relative to each other. This instability manifests itself as a susceptibility to attack by atmospheric oxygen. The consequence of this is that products which contain significant amounts of unsaturated fat are liable to develop flavour taints if not protected. Butter, for example, will deteriorate rapidly if left accidently in sunlight, which acts catalytically.

In the simplest terms, fat consists of a mixture of glycerides, and a glyceride is a compound of glycerol and fatty acids. There is a wide range of naturally occurring fatty acids, though some are commoner than others. This makes for a variety of glycerides, and for fats, that vary from source to source.

Glycerol is a trihydric alcohol, $\text{CH}_2\text{OH.CHOH.CH}_2\text{OH}$, each hydroxyl (OH) of which is joined to a fatty acid to form a triglyceride. The process of combination is known as esterification. If only one hydroxyl is esterified a monoglyceride is formed, if two, a diglyceride. We will meet these two kinds of compounds later when we come to consider emulsifiers.

Fatty acids consist of a paraffinic chain coupled to a carboxylic group, COOH, and the commonest unsaturated acid is oleic acid, $\text{CH}_3(\text{CH}_2)_7\text{CH}=\text{CH}(\text{CH}_2)_7\text{COOH}$ with just one double bond, but there are acids with two, three, or four double bonds to be found in plant and animal fats, and even more in fats from fish. One plant acid of particular biological importance to humans is linoleic acid, $\text{CH}_3(\text{CH}_2)_4(\text{CH}=\text{CHCH}_2)_2(\text{CH}_2)_6$ COOH, that is, with two specifically sited double bonds. It is called an essential fatty acid because, although the body needs it, a key enzyme for making it is missing from the body, and so the acid must be present in the fat of the diet. So, quite apart from the hazard of taint formation, this acid must be protected from oxidation because linoleic acid is a precursor within the body of two physiologically important acids: γ-linolenic acid: $CH_3(CH_2)_4$ $(CH=CHCH_2)_3(CH_2)_3COOH$ with three double bonds; arachidonic acid: $CH_3(CH_2)_4(CH=CHCH_2)_4(CH_2)_4COOH$ with four double bonds.

Arachidonic acid is needed for the lipid component of biological membranes, lipid being a generic term applied to all fatty compounds, of which glycerides form a coherent subgroup. In membrane lipids one of the glycerol hydroxyls is esterified to a phosphoric acid grouping of one sort or another (see section on emulsifiers) to provide a hydrophilic/hydrophobic structure necessary to membrane stability.[16] It is not certain whether linoleic acid is converted to arachidonic acid within the membrane or prior to that. *In situ* it is protected by the natural antioxidant, tocopherol, which will be discussed later.

Apart from that, both arachidonic acid and γ-linolenic acid are precursors for prostaglandins, mysterious substances which, in some way, play a part in the functioning of smooth muscle, that is, muscle associated with hollow organs such as blood vessels and the gut.

So far as food is concerned, therefore, protection must be given to the unsaturated fat it contains, not only because of the noxious taints that could otherwise develop, but also because of the loss of valuable essential fatty acid that would follow. It is implicit in this, of course, that the diet should be arranged to contain sufficient essential fatty acid.

In order to understand how antioxidants work, something must first be said of how oxidation proceeds. It may be noted, in passing, that small amounts of metals, such as copper and iron, act as catalysts in the mechanisms now to be described, and an essential step in any refining treatment of fats is to remove such metals as far as possible. We will come back to this when discussing sequestrants. Paradoxically, as we shall see later, certain trace elements are necessary to a balanced diet and that will be discussed in due course.

Oxidation proceeds in two stages, initiation and propagation. Initiation involves the formulation of a free radical—that is, a compound made unstable and reactive by the removal of a hydrogen *atom*—at one or other of the carbon atoms adjacent to a double bond. There can then be interchange as shown below to produce a total of four free radicals.[17]

$$-CH^*-CH=CH-CH_2- \qquad -CH_2-CH=CH-CH^*-$$

$$\Updownarrow \qquad \text{and} \qquad \Updownarrow$$

$$-CH^*-CH=CH-CH_2- \qquad -CH_2-CH^*-CH=CH-$$

In the absence of antioxidant, propagation will proceed in two stages: first a peroxide being formed and then a new free radical produced:

$$-CH^*-CH=CH-CH_2- \; + \; O_2 \longrightarrow \; -\underset{\underset{O-O^*}{|}}{CH}-CH=CH-CH_2-$$

$$-\underset{\underset{O-O^*}{|}}{CH}-CH=CH-CH_2- \; + \; -CH_2-CH=CH- \longrightarrow$$

$$-\underset{\underset{O-OH}{|}}{CH}-CH=CH-CH_2- \; + \; -CH^*-CH=CH-$$

Similar reactions occur with the other free radicals. The hydroperoxides that are formed are unstable and break down to smaller carbonyl—that is, aldehydic or ketonic—substances. For example, one of the breakdown patterns of oleic acid would be:

$$CH_3(CH_2)_7CH=CH(CH_2)_7COOH \; + \; O_2 \longrightarrow$$
$$CH_3(CH_2)_7CHO \; + \; OCH(CH_2)_7COOH$$

It is such substances that are responsible for flavour taint and some can produce this when present at a level of less than 1 part per million. It is the function of antioxidants to intervene before significant radical propagation takes place.

Without intervention the chain reaction would terminate only by fortuitous interaction of free radicals. A good antioxidant will mop up the free radicals as they are formed. It has been the job of food scientists to devise substances that were both effective and safe, but though theoretical considerations readily lead one to a promising class of substances, selection of the most suitable for a set of circumstances is more of an empirical exercise, albeit a systematic one: quite apart from toxicological testing.

Looking at the list of permitted antioxidants set out below, it will be obvious to those versed in photographic techniques that some have their origins there. Indeed, long before any serious work had been done on antioxidants in food products, or vitamins had been added to any of them, it had been the habit to stabilize preparations of fat-soluble vitamins with hydroquinone. More acceptable substances have since been adopted, but during the long years of investigation no rat seems to have suffered from the hydroquinone it absorbed, nor did those of us who acted as human guinea pigs in the cause of progress.

In the event, greater interest has developed in the gallates, or rather in fat-soluble derivatives of them, and in two other substituted phenolic compounds, butylated hydroxytoluene and butylated hydroxyanisole (the butyl group here providing fat solublization): while those looking to more natural sources have investigated the tocopherols and fat-soluble derivatives of ascorbic acid. We shall meet both of these later in other roles: tocopherol as vitamin E and ascorbic acid as vitamin C. The acid itself is water soluble and so can be used directly in beverages as an antioxidant.

It is indicative of the problems that beset those concerned with rules and regulations that ascorbic acid appeared in the U.K. list of approved antioxidants only when the U.K. became a member of the EEC. Previously, having been accepted as a vitamin, it did not need regulating for another purpose.

We will use the U.K. list as illustrative of general practice, though it lacks one substance, nordihydroguaiaretic acid, that appears in other lists; this because it is U.K. practice not to admit substances which it is considered not to be any better than others already in the list. Other countries are prepared to admit any substance that is proven to be safe. The U.K. list[18] is:

Butylated hydroxytoluene(BHT)	Calcium L-ascorbate
Butylated hydroxyanisole (BHA)	Ascorbyl palmitate
	(6-O-palmityl-L-ascorbate)
Propyl gallate	Natural tocopherol extract
Octyl gallate	Synthetic α-tocopherol
Dodecyl gallate	Synthetic β-tocopherol
L-Ascorbic acid	Synthetic δ-tocopherol
Sodium L-ascorbate	Ethoxyquin

ANTIOXIDANTS

Butylated hydroxytoluene(BHT)
2,6-di-t-butyl-4-methylphenol

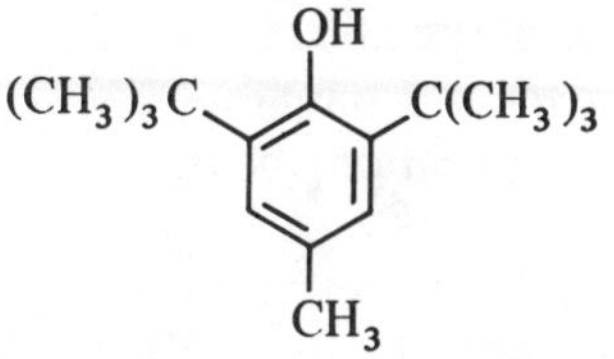

Butylated hydroxyanisole(BHA)
mixture of 2- and 3-t-butyl-4-
hydroxyanisole

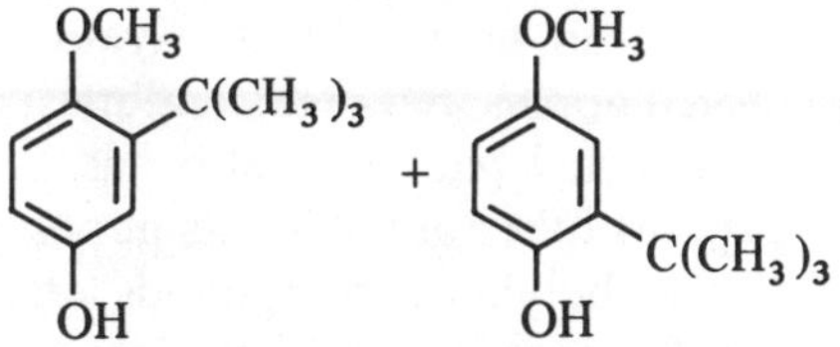

Propyl gallate

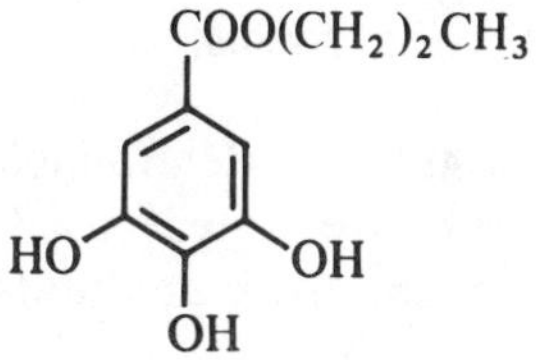

Octyl gallate

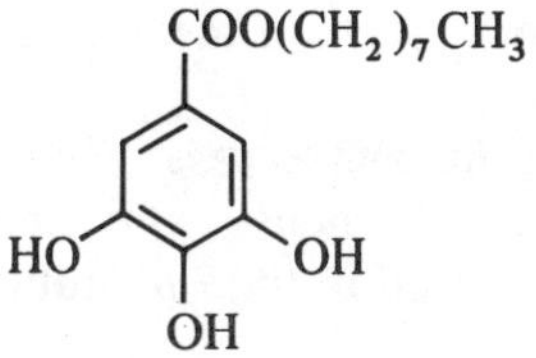

Dodecyl gallate

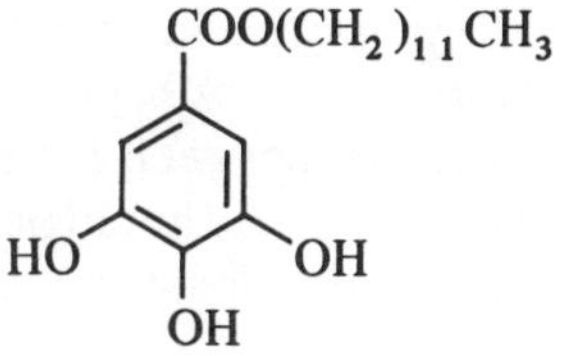

Antioxidants (*continued*)

L-Ascorbic Acid (vitamin C)	Sodium L-ascorbate	Ascorbyl palmitate

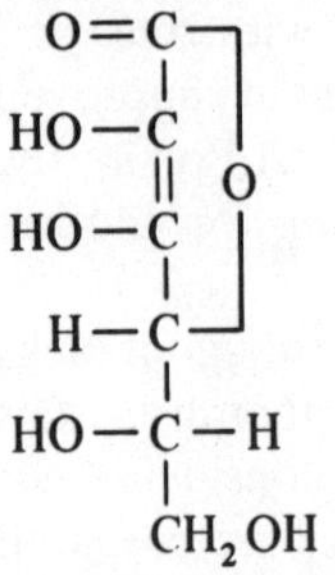

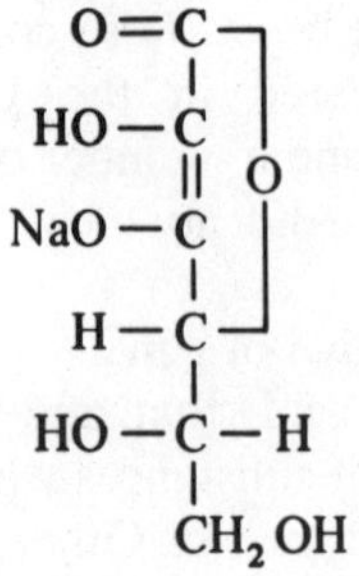

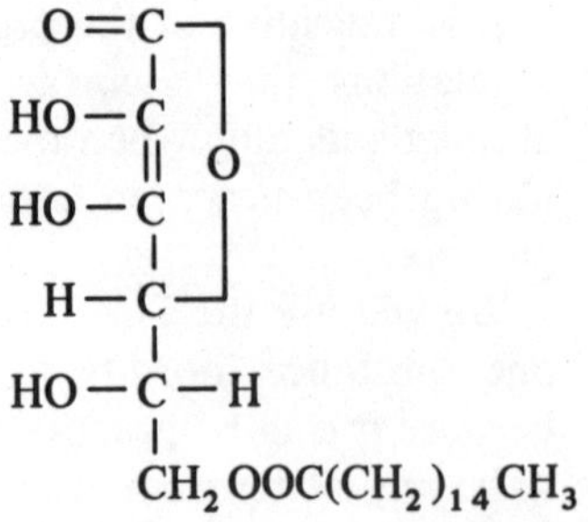

Tocopherol—R^1, R^2, and R^3 may be either H or CH_3, α-tocopherol, which is also vitamin E—$R^1 = R^2 = R^3 = CH_3$.

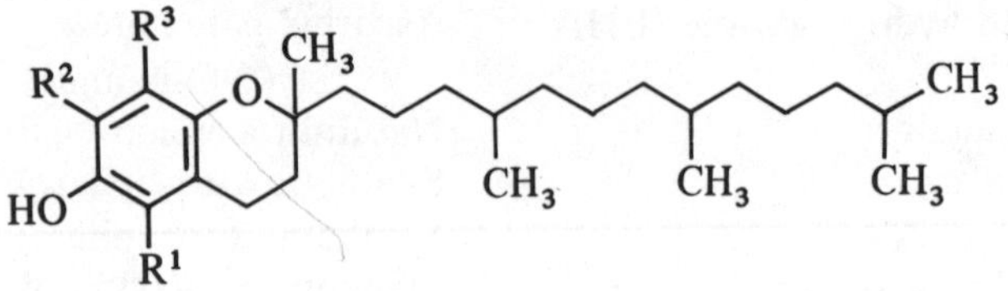

Ethoxyquin

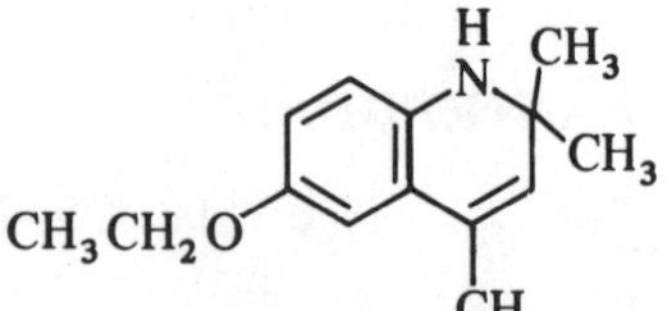

We can deal with ethoxyquin quickly. It has a specific application to stored apples and pears and must not exceed a level of 3 p.p.m.

Ascorbyl palmitate also has a rather limited application, being used to support other antioxidants in polyphase food systems.

The butylated compounds and the gallates are very effective but are strictly controlled. They are not permitted in baby foods. Neither the tocopherol nor the ascorbic acid compounds have any restrictions on use beyond that determined by good manufacturing practice and tocopherols replace the phenolic compounds in baby foods. Ascorbic acid compounds are preferred for moist foods, such as meat and bakery products, and for liquids, such as beer.

Choice between the phenolic compounds, where permitted, is determined solely by technological requirements and mixtures are often used. Application is limited to fats used in food manufacture, and there are limits of addition according to the kind of antioxidant and the kind of fat. Thus edible fats may contain up to 200 mg/kg of BHT or BHA, or any mixture of them, and up to 100 mg/kg of any gallate or mixture of them.

Both BHT and BHA are permitted in potato flour, flakes or granules to a maximum of 25 mg/kg, and BHT in chewing gum up to 200 mg/kg.

The FAO/WHO list[19] a number of derivative compounds not in the U.K. list, as well as nordihydroguaiaretic acid.

Preservatives

Preservatives are often grouped with antioxidants because both classes of additives serve to protect food from spoilage. But whereas antioxidants are used to limit oxidative spoilage, particularly of fats, preservatives aim to prevent microbial spoilage, which can affect not only the fat contained in the food, but also the protein. The World Health Organization has estimated that some 20% of the world's food supply is lost through this kind of spoilage[13] and this is very serious indeed.

Protection of food against spoilage of this kind has been a preoccupation of mankind ever since food resources began to be organized many centuries ago. Drying was one of the earliest, if not the earliest form of protection, to be followed in due course by salt pickling, vinegar pickling, and smoking. These are the traditional methods of protection still in use today, but, no matter how attractive the preserved food might be in its own right—and some are still popular—they are somewhat different foods from the raw commodity so far as the human palate is concerned. So there have been more modern processes—canning, dehydration (which is not the same as drying), and quick freezing—which aim to retain as much of the original character of the food as possible. Canning, however, can be used only for foods that are to be eaten in cooked form, and often some supplementary preservative is needed. The other two are relatively expensive processes, that have to provide some particular advantage for which the consumer is prepared to pay. In quick freezing, for example, it is a greater retention of out-of-season freshness. But there are many run-of-the-mill foods, such as jams, fruit extracts, cheeses, cured meats, and so on, that pass through retail shops daily and require some simple *in situ* protection.

It is interesting to observe that needs have been met by a relatively short basic list of compounds, thirteen in fact, though derivatives, offering some technological advantage or other, raise the total to 34.[20] No fine theories can be presented to indicate a line of attack when searching for suitable preservatives, but the search has not been wholly empiric. It has been based more on intelligent, albeit accidental, observations.

That has not stopped people looking for clues that would support postulated mechanisms, of which there are currently three.[21] One is interference with the cell membrane of the invading microorganism; the second, interference with genetic mechanisms; and the third, interference with intracellular enzymic activity. Insofar as suitable and acceptable substances have been found, however, there is no great incentive to establish a theoretical case, and it is unlikely that the matter will be pursued with any great vigour.

The emergence of nisin as a preservative is typical of this observational empiricism. It is a short polypeptide containing seven amino acids, and it is now recognized as an antibiotic that is particularly active against clostridia and lactobacillae. It is a natural component of some cheeses and is therefore an obvious choice as preservative for other cheeses. It is now used also in canned foods that are prone to clostridial spoilage.

With sodium nitrate/nitrate we have another case of fortuitous observation, though the benefit is still a matter of continued discussion. Crude rock salt, used in earlier days to preserve meat, was observed to produce pink patches on occasion, and these patches were found to be due to the contaminant sodium nitrate, which was reduced to the nitrite by resident microorganisms. This in turn reacted with muscle myoglobin to produce the red colouring. So nitrate, or nitrite, was then added to produce a uniformly attractive colour. One may argue about the ethics of this, but there was a wholly unexpected bonus, for the additive was found to be highly effective in preventing the growth of *Clostridium botulinum*, a dangerous pathogen that must be continuously guarded against. Unfortunately, in exerting its preservative action, nitrite itself is liable to be converted to nitrosoamine, which is a carcinogen, and there is a risk/benefit situation. The preservative action is so good that the substance cannot be lightly abandoned, and the present situation is that addition is limited to a level that minimizes the chance of carcinogenic action while remaining effective against botulinum. Meanwhile a search for an effective alternative proceeds.

The principal basic preservatives are as follows:

Benzoic acid	C_6H_5COOH
Methyl 4-hydroxybenzoate	$HOC_6H_4COOCH_3$
Ethyl 4-hydroxybenzoate	$HOC_6H_4COOC_2H_5$
Propyl 4-hydroxybenzoate	$HOC_6H_4COOC_3H_7$
Sodium nitrate	$NaNO_3$
Sodium nitrite	$NaNO_2$
Propionic acid	C_2H_5COOH
Sorbic acid	$CH_3CH=CHCH=CH-COOH$
Sulphur dioxide	SO_2

Of these the most commonly used is sulphur dioxide (or compounds that release it, such as the sulphites). It is permitted in 52 kinds of food. Benzoic acid, or one of its derivatives, is permitted in 24 kinds of food; but it should be kept in mind that, according to published work,[22,23] the benzoates can promote an allergic response in sensitive people.

Sulphur dioxide and benzoic acid act as bacteriocides and the preference, as shown above, is for sulphur dioxide. But this is pungent and it is not always advisable to use it for this reason. It is also sometimes difficult to incorporate. Sorbic acid is a fungistat and so is more effective against moulds and yeasts. It is a permitted additive to drinks like cider, wine, and perry. It may also be used in nut pastes, prunes, cheese, and flour confectionery. However it has not yet been checked as exhaustively as the authorities would like and its use is still being monitored.

The presence of propionic acid in the list is unusual and interesting: and a prime example of empirical action. It is a short-chain acid of unusual occurrence. Most naturally occurring fatty acids have an even number of carbon atoms in their molecular structure, but this one has three. It is produced commonly by bacterial metabolism and, in fact, is so produced in the rumen of cattle and thereby finds its way into butterfat. It is permitted in bread, flour confectionery—and Christmas puddings, and probably acts as a fungistat. If it has any bactericidal action, it can be only by interfering with propionic acid activity by the bacteria.

Emulsifiers and Stabilizers

Any substance which is capable of aiding the formation of a stable mixture of two otherwise immiscible substances, for example, fat and water, is called an emulsifier; and any substance that helps to maintain an emulsion when it has been formed is called a stabilizer. The stabilizer may have the same basic characteristic as an emulsifier, or it may serve to thicken one or other participant of the emulsion, or make it more viscous and hence less likely to separate into its components. Such substances are widely used in the commercial production of bread, flour confectionery, ice cream, margarine, chocolate, and sugar confectionery.[24]

Foods need emulsifiers because all of them, whether natural or manufactured, contain water as well as the three main nutrient constituents, proteins, carbohydrates, and fats. Natural foods have their own inbuilt emulsifier systems. In fact this holds for all living organisms and they are an essential part of the whole life system. Some of them are extracted for use in manufactured food. Other emulsifiers mimic natural emulsifiers, but others again rely on first principles for fabrication. The principle of an emulsifier is that it should have within its molecular structure one grouping with an affinity for water and another with an affinity for fat.

Let us look at this in some detail, starting with the terms miscible and immiscible. Water and methanol, CH_3OH, are miscible in all proportions, which is to say that each will dissolve in the other. So will water and ethanol, CH_3CH_2OH. We can generalize the whole family of such alcohols as $CH_3(CH_2)_nOH$, where $CH_3(CH_2)_n-$ is a water-hating paraffinic chain and $-OH$ is a water-loving group. (If we write water as $H-OH$ we see why this should be.) We call the one hydrophobic and the other hydrophilic.

The reason why methanol and ethanol are soluble is that the power of the OH group to attract another is greater than the repulsion between it and a short paraffinic chain. But as the length of the chain increases, so the power of repulsion grows until the chain is pushed out. Nevertheless the attraction between the OH of water and that of the alcohol remains and the alcohol is anchored to the surface of the water. If that surface is now covered, either with a film of paraffin or one of liquid oil, the alcohol chains will be dissolved in it and so produce cohesion between the two surfaces. This is a very simplified introduction but what we have is a two-phase system and, when it is stirred, one phase will break up into small globules and disperse in the other. This is an emulsion and the long-chain alcohol is acting as the emulsifier.

Which one breaks up depends on a number of factors that do not concern us here, but the importance of them is well illustrated by the making of butter from cream. In cream the fat phase is dispersed as globules in the serum. That is to say, it is a fat-in-water emulsion. It contains about 30% fat. Each globule is surrounded by a membrane which serves as emulsifier. Like all biological membranes, it contains both lipid and protein and is known as a lipoprotein. We have seen earlier that a membrane itself depends for its stability on a hydrophilic/hydrophobic structure. Now we have to conceive an extension to this idea in that the membrane can be so aligned that it presents a majority of hydrophilic groups on one side and hydrophobic groups on the other, the hydrophilic groups now being of a proteinaceous character.

When the cream is churned, the lipoprotein skin is broken, the balance is disturbed and the fat globules coalesce. Now phosphatides take over the role of emulsifier. Much of the aqueous part comes away as whey, but the remainder, comprising some 18% of the remaining fat/water mixture is trapped as the water-in-fat emulsion we call butter. This is known as phase inversion.

Phosphatides are a class of naturally occurring substances—some related to the glycerides—that are widely involved in biological systems when two immiscible phases have to be kept in close proximity. When they first came under scientific scrutiny, they were called lecithins and the name is still in use today. Soya bean lecithin, for example, is one of the most commonly used emulsifiers. In general, however, it refers to a commercial preparation of mixed character. Let us now put the phosphatides into context.

Following on from our discussion of triglycerides in the section on antioxidants, let us formulate a simple triglyceride thus:

$$
\begin{array}{l}
CH_2OOCR^1 \\
\quad | \\
R^2COOCH \\
\quad | \\
CH_2OOCR^3
\end{array}
$$

where R^1, R^2, and R^3 are the paraffinic chains, $CH_3(CH_2)_n-$, of the fatty acid radicals. Suppose we now remove two of the radicals. We are left with a monoglyceride:

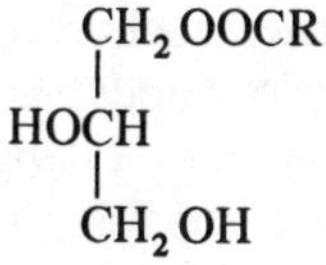

$$
\begin{array}{l}
CH_2OOCR^1 \\
| \\
HOCH \\
| \\
CH_2OH
\end{array}
$$

This will act as an emulsifier because of the two hydrophilic OH groups and the hydrophobic R^1 group. If only one of the radicals had been removed there would have been a diglyceride with weaker emulsifying powers. By varying the proportions of mono- and diglycerides in a mixture and selecting the fats to provide preferred values of R, a range of emulsifiers can be prepared.

In practice, fatty acid radicals are not so much removed as reorganized. Thus for example, if a fat is refluxed with an equimolecular quantity of glycerol, we get:

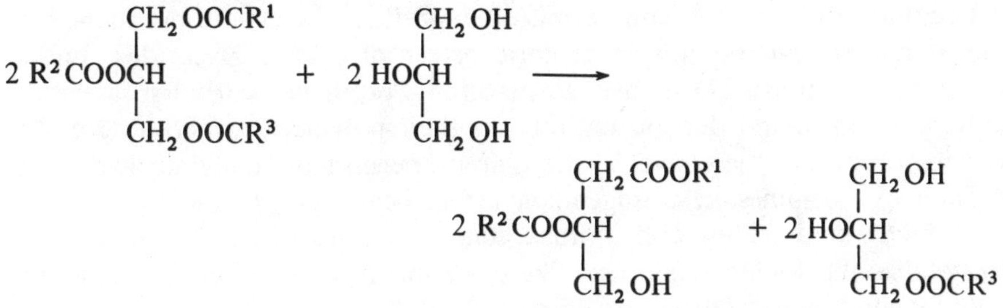

$$
2\ \begin{array}{l} CH_2OOCR^1 \\ | \\ R^2COOCH \\ | \\ CH_2OOCR^3 \end{array}
\quad + \quad
2\ \begin{array}{l} CH_2OH \\ | \\ HOCH \\ | \\ CH_2OH \end{array}
\quad \longrightarrow
$$

$$
2\ \begin{array}{l} CH_2COOR^1 \\ | \\ R^2COOCH \\ | \\ CH_2OH \end{array}
\quad + \quad
2\ \begin{array}{l} CH_2OH \\ | \\ HOCH \\ | \\ CH_2OOCR^3 \end{array}
$$

Mono and diglycerides are then separated by molecular distillation.

Suppose now that we were to replace one of the fatty acid radicals of a triglyceride with a phosphoric acid radical. We would obtain a phospholipid, or phosphatide, of the general form:

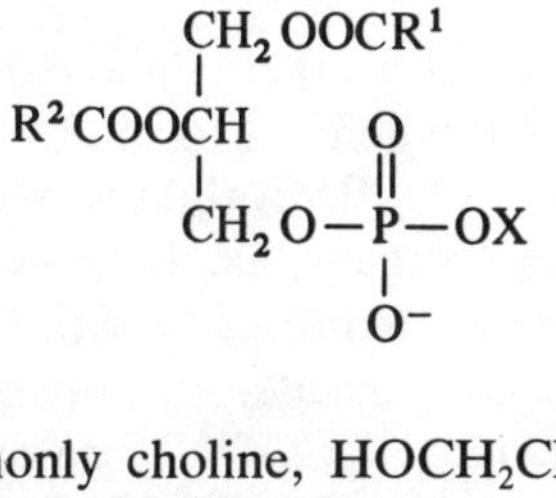

$$
\begin{array}{l}
CH_2OOCR^1 \\
| \\
R^2COOCH \qquad\ \ O \\
| \qquad\qquad\quad\ \, \| \\
CH_2O-P-OX \\
\qquad\qquad\ | \\
\qquad\qquad\ O^-
\end{array}
$$

In this OX is most commonly choline, $HOCH_2CH_2OHN(CH_3)_3$, and less commonly, ethanolamine, $HOCH_2CH_2NH_2$.

The lecithins[16] include both compounds. All forms of phospholipids have been isolated and identified, but separation is not easy and commercial lecithins are mixtures whose exact composition is not known. Even ammonium phosphatides, used in chocolate making, whose title might suggest a known composition, are described as 'essentially a mixture of ammonium salts of phosphatidic acids derived from partially hardened rapeseed oil together with unreacted partially hardened rapeseed oil.' (For the uninitiated, hardening is a process whereby the degree of unsaturation of a fat, i.e. the number of double bonds, is reduced by interaction with hydrogen.) Such a product is a consequence of expertise in which the emulsifying properties are shaped to satisfy the technological requirements of the product.

Indeed this could be said of a number of the emulsifiers in the permitted list. Thus we find partial glycerides esterified with acetic acid (CH_3COOH), lactic acid ($CH_3CHOHCOOH$), citric acid ($CH_2COOH.HOCCOOH.CH_2COOH$) or diacetyltartaric acid ($COOH.HCOOCCH_3HCOOCCH_3.COOH$). It is doubtful if any *a priori* reasoning led to their synthesis, yet we find them in use in the breadmaking industry, and perfectly safe to use. One suspects them to work more as stabilizers than emulsifiers, for the esters will lack any strong hydrophilic action. And similarly for sodium and calcium stearoyl lactylate where the hydroxyl group (OH) is blocked by esterification with stearic acid.

Lecithins are also the main permitted emulsifiers for cheese products, but the stabilizers are no longer esoteric esters of partial glycerides, but a selection of gums. These are all naturally occurring carbohydrates, or polysaccharides, and depend entirely on their polymeric structures for the varying properties they have. Those that are permitted are alginic acid or its sodium or calcium salt, carrageenan, locust bean gum, tragacanth, acacia, ghatti gum, karaya gum, and xanthan gum. These are all viscous gums, used to stabilize the system. Their use, like those incorporated in bread, is limited only by good manufacturing practice.

There is one group of emulsifiers that can be claimed to be original in design. They are based on three groups of compounds—polyoxyethylenes, sorbitans, and fatty acids—and, by varying the composition, a very wide range of properties can be produced. They may include all three, or exclude polyoxyethylene or sorbitan.

Polyoxyethylene is produced from ethylene oxide $-CH_2-CH_2-$ by a free radical reaction, and it has the general formula $-(OCH_2CH_2)_nOH$, where n is commonly of the order of 20. Sorbitans are dehydration products of the naturally occurring sugar alcohol, sorbitol. They and the polyoxyethylenes can be esterified directly with fatty acids, and the sorbitan esters may themselves be condensed with polyoxyethylene. The fatty acids that are used are lauric ($C_{11}H_{23}COOH$), palmitic ($C_{15}H_{31}COOH$), oleic ($C_{17}H_{33}COOH$), and stearic ($C_{17}H_{35}COOH$). It needs little imagination to appreciate the variation in composition, and hence of behaviour, that is possible.

There are 57 substances in all in the U.K. permitted list,[25] plus two that

EMULSIFIERS

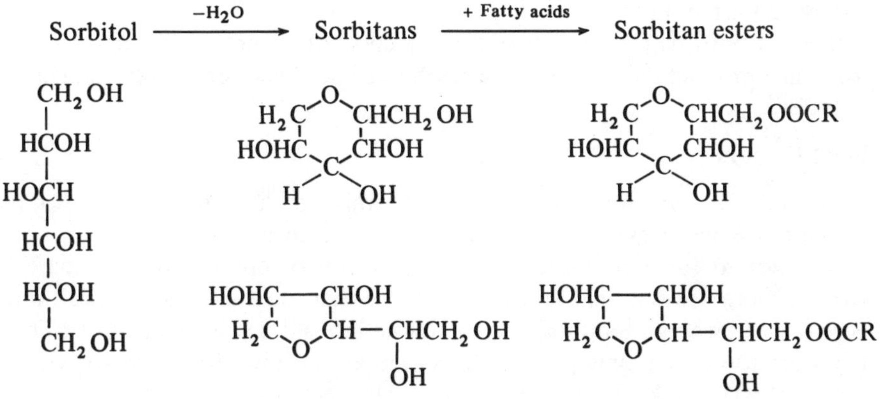

Sorbitol $\xrightarrow{-H_2O}$ Sorbitans $\xrightarrow{\text{+ Fatty acids}}$ Sorbitan esters

Sorbitans condensed with ethylene oxide ⟶ polyoxyethylenesorbitans
(These compounds can be further reacted with fatty acids if required.)

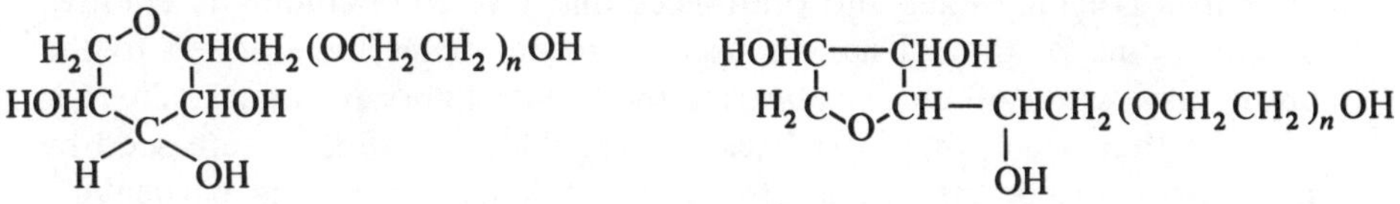

Quillaia

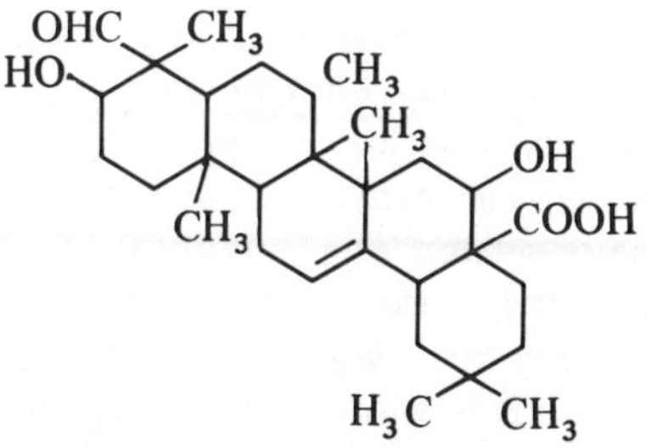

are no more than tin-greasing compounds and are relevant only insofar as
they may seep into the product. That so many are permitted is a measure of
technological requirements since, according to U.K. ruling, no substance is
admitted if an already admitted substance is doing the job adequately. One
that is so unique as to be quite outside a general discussion of emulsifiers is
quillaia, an extract of a South American tree bark, a time-honoured additive
to soft drinks to produce a head of foam. Its active principle is a saponin. A
saponin is so-called because it is akin to soap in its ability to foam, but the
similarity ends there. They are complex materials in which the hydrophobic

moiety is provided either by a steroid grouping or, as in quillaia, a triterpenoid grouping. The hydrophilic moiety is built up from monosaccharide units.

Apart from this odd-man-out, the selection of an emulsifier or stabilizer for a new product will be seen as a matter of both experience and expertise.

Food Colours

Colour plays an important role in all walks of life and in many of its activities. When present in food it can be both attractive and pleasing, but this is not to say that there is any uniformity of opinion on the matter. Indeed there are national likes and dislikes that must always be taken into account. So, when a food process, desirable in itself, leads to a loss of colour from the food, or a new product looks unduly insipid, the processor wisely takes steps to make it more attractive. The fact that the steps taken may vary from country to country does not imply that one knows better than another, but rather that likes and prejudices vary. Indeed it is likely that arguments on food colours have done more to cloud objective assessment of additives as a whole than that on any other class.

For it is not only likes and prejudices that give food colour its emotive content. Some of the substances used in recent times have added to the controversy, with coal tar dyes bearing the brunt of abrasive attack. There is no doubt that, when they first became available, the colours were seen by manufacturers to be the solution to all their colouring problems, particularly as such minute quantities were required to provide a suitable depth of colour. Unfortunately, it would have been impossible at the time to apply the right kind of critical judgement, for the toxicological knowledge was lacking that would have permitted it. And there were no evident reactions to suggest that they presented any kind of hazard at the very low levels of addition. Indeed hazard was not envisaged.

Present controversy is a consequence of the recognition of cancer as a major—if not the major—cause of premature disease and death, and of a wide-ranging search for the causes of cancer. Dyestuffs are suspect, and the most suspect have already been winkled out. It matters not that there are substances present naturally in food that are more hazardous than any in the currently permitted list of dyestuffs, the winkling will continue as tests become more refined and more acceptable colouring substances are evolved. In the meantime, since it is as much a matter of judgement as of scientific assessment, the winkling has been uneven between one country and another.

The basis of colour is relatively easy to understand. We have already explained what double bonds in an organic compound are, and a glance at the formulae for food colours will show that each contains many double bonds. And there is system in the arrangement, for each double bond alternates with a single bond. This is called a conjugated system and its effect is to cause an arrangement of electrons within the molecule that is sensitive to incident light. White light is compounded of red, orange, yellow, green, blue, indigo, and violet light. It is called a spectrum of colour and, according to the system of conjugation present in the molecule, one or other part of the spectrum will be absorbed and removed from the spectrum. The residual colour depends on which part of the spectrum has been absorbed. There are other methods of producing colour, but dyestuffs were a consequence of understanding this method and applying it.

The FAO/WHO (see Chapter 5) in their most recent deliberations on food colours[37] have said of dyestuffs that up-to-date toxicological evaluation (see Chapter 6) would require minimum data as follows: metabolic studies with several species of animal, including man: covering absorption, distribution, biotransformation, and elimination: with attempts to identify metabolic products at each step. There should also be short-term feeding studies on a non-rodent mammalian species, multigeneration reproduction/teratogenicity studies, and long-term carcinogenic/toxicity studies in two species of animals (see Chapter 6). It would also like to see introduced chromatographic analyses for the purpose of specification. American authorities have calculated that it would take four years to carry out such a programme on just eight of their provisionally approved list of dyestuffs.

On the subject of natural colours the report presents the view that naturalness *per se* does not assure safety, though it accepts that 'a colour isolated in a chemically unmodified form from a recognized foodstuff and used in the foodstuff from which it is extracted at levels normally found in that food' would provide a product as acceptable 'as the food itself with no requirement for biological testing.' Why anyone should wish to go through this extraordinary procedure is puzzling, albeit indicative of the furore that the campaign against colour additives has produced. The report adds that the extracted colour would require tests if it were to be put back into food at a higher level, or put into another food, or chemically modified after extraction, or if it had been extracted from a non-food source.

The report recognizes a problem in specifying natural colour preparations when geographical, geological, and climatic conditions—and the method of isolation—may determine overall composition. Nevertheless, it has to admit that such 'preparations have been used in food over a long period of time and have been accepted for use without supporting toxicological evidence in much the same manner as vegetable and cereal products.' This of course is a challenge for all safety testing. Why should the toxicant risks of additives be pursued so much more rigorously than those of some common foods?. It is this author's view that nature-identical substances, properly purified, are generally to be preferred to an extract of the natural material.

There are 31 dyestuffs on the FAO/WHO list of evaluated substances,[19] but a number of these have had qualifications attached to their use. There were 31 in the 1960 U.K. list, but the two lists differed considerably, as Table 3 shows. Thirteen of the U.K. colours were withdrawn between 1960

Table 3. Dyestuff Food Colours

FAO/WHO list: as at May 1977 (many with conditional use)	U.K. list: 1960	U.K. list: added by 1975
Acid Fuchsine FB	Amaranth	Black 7984**
Allura Red AC	Azorubine	Brilliant Blue FCF***
Amaranth	Brilliant Black BN	Fast Yellow AB**
Azorubine (Carmoisine)	Blue VRS*	Patent Blue V
Brilliant Black BN	(t) Brown FK***	Indanthrene Blue RS**
Brilliant Blue FCF	Chocolate Brown FB***	
Brown FK	(t) Chocolate Brown HT***	*Japanese list: 1977*
Chocolate Brown HT	Erythrosine BS	Acid Red
Chrysoine	Fast Red E*	Amaranth****
Eosin	Green S	Brilliant Blue FCF
Erythrosine	Indigo Carmine	Erythrosine****
Fast Green FCF	Naphthol Yellow S*	Fast Green FCF
Fast Red E	Oil Yellow GG*	Indigo Carmine
Fast Yellow AB	Oil Yellow XP*	Phloxine
Green S	Orange G***	Ponceau 4R****
Indanthrene (Solanthrene) Blue RS	Orange RN**	Rose Bengale
Indigo Carmine (Indigotine)	Ponceau MX*	Sunset Yellow FCF
Patent Blue V	Ponceau SX*	Tartrazine
Ponceau 4R	Ponceau 3R*	
Ponceau 6R	Ponceau 4R	
Quinoline Yellow	Quinoline Yellow	
Red 2G	(t) Red 2G***	
Red 10B	Red 6B*	
Scarlet GN	Red 10B*	
Sudan G	Red FB*	
Sudan Red G	Sunset Yellow FCF	
Sunset Yellow FCF	Tartrazine	
Tartrazine	Violet BNP	
Violet 5BN	Yellow 2G***	
Yellow 2G	Yellow RFS*	
Yellow 27175N	Yellow RY*	

*Colours removed from UK list by 1975.
**Colours removed in 1976.
***Colours not in EEC list, but with 3 years temporary permit if marked (t).
****Current voluntary ban on use.

and 1972[26] and another one by 1976. Five other dyestuffs were admitted to the U.K. list by 1975, but 3 of them had disappeared again by 1976, leaving a residue of 20 permitted dyestuffs. Seven of them, however, are not in the EEC approved list and will presumably disappear as harmonization proceeds. Five of the 7, in fact, have a three-year temporary use limitation placed on them. By way of contrast, the Japanese list only 11 colours,[27] of which 8 appear in the FAO/WHO list: but of these 8 the Japanese have placed a temporary ban on 3. India[28] has a list of just 10 colours, all of which are in the FAO/WHO list.

SOME DYESTUFF FOOD COLOURS IN CURRENT USE

Note that the basis of colour is a conjugated system in which double bonds alternate with single bonds. N atoms in the system intensify colour.

Amaranth

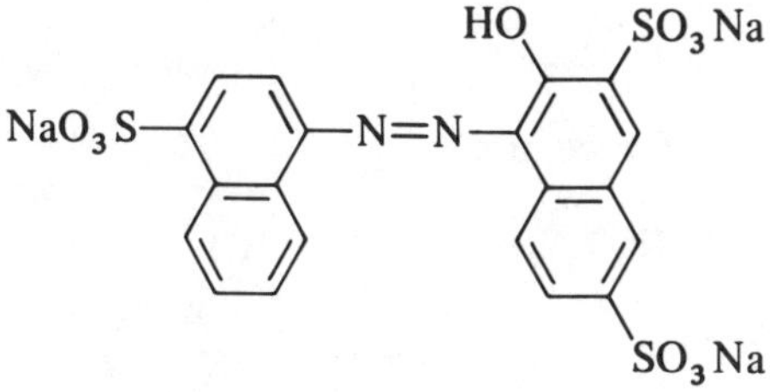

Erythrosine BS

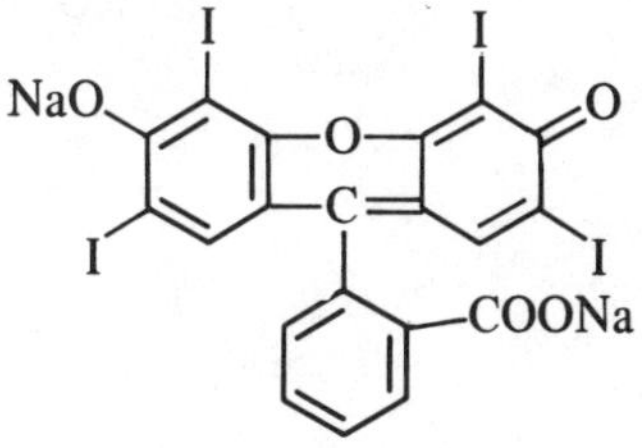

Azorubine

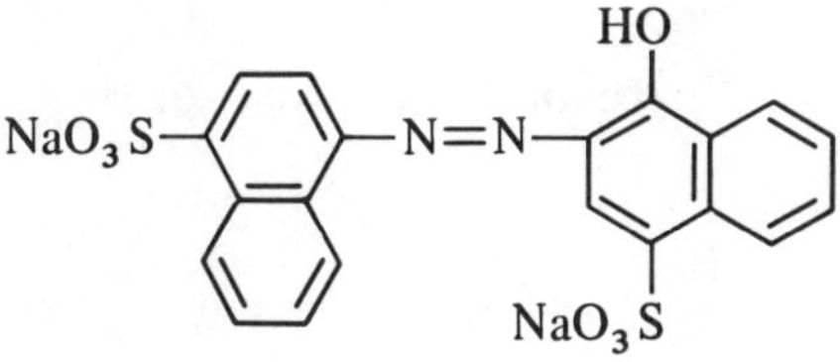

Green S

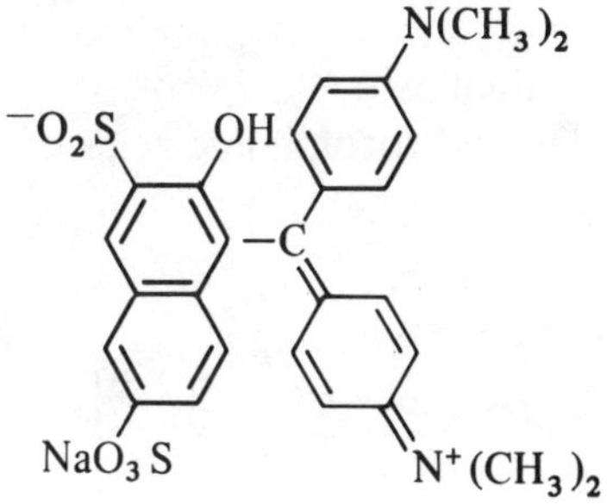

Brilliant Black BN

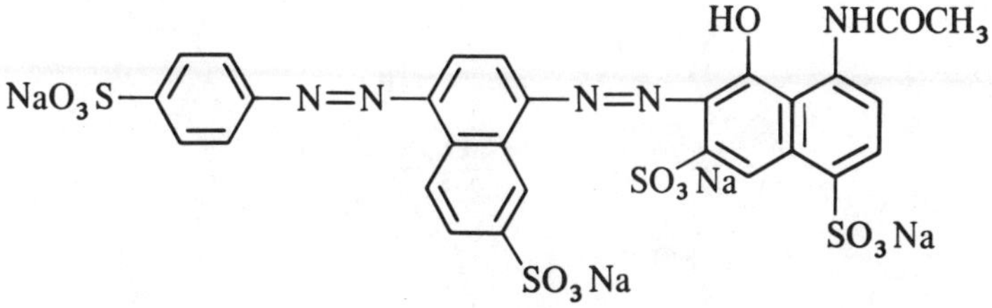

Indigo Carmine

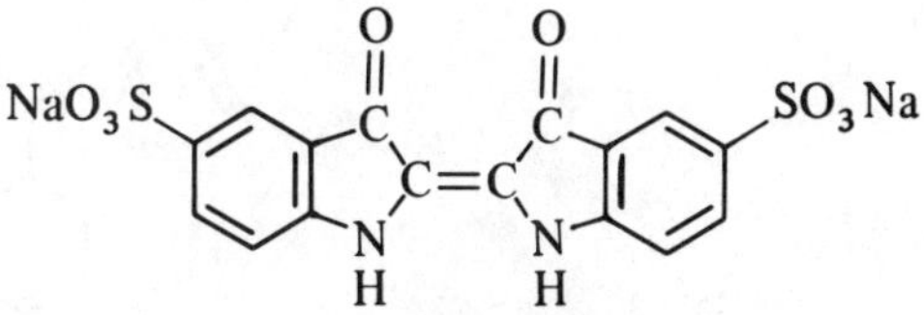

Some Dyestuff Food Colours in Current Use (*continued*)

Chocolate Brown HT

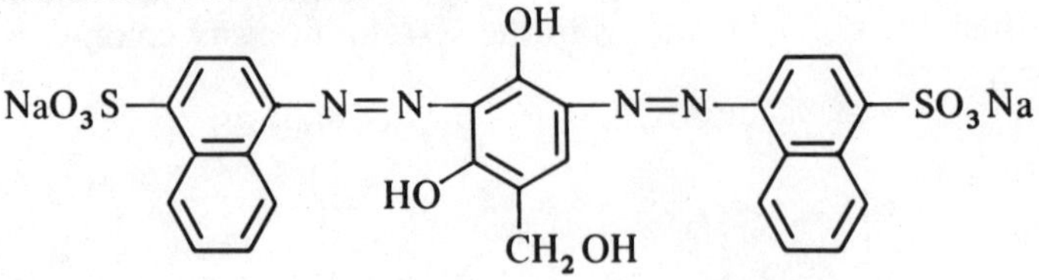

Ponceau 4R

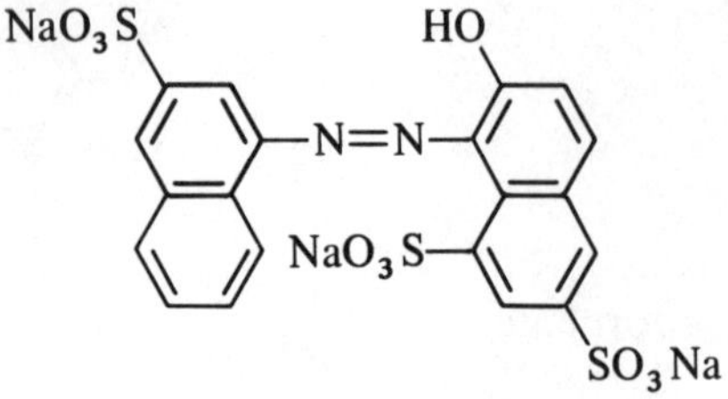

Quinoline Yellow
Di- and trisulphonic acids of a mixture of 2 parts of A and 1 part of B

A

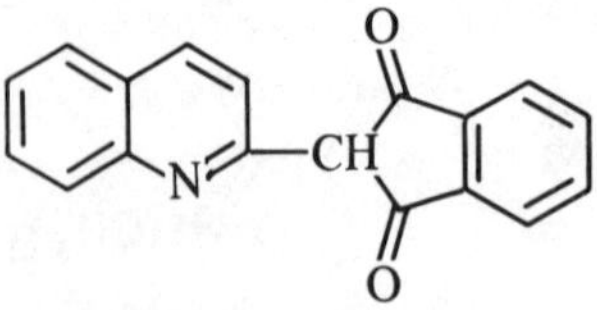

B

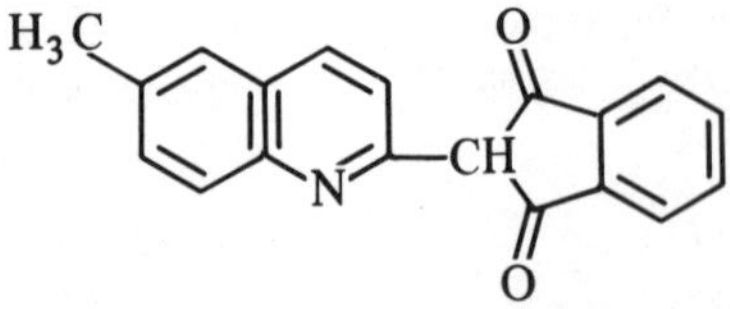

Sunset Yellow FCF

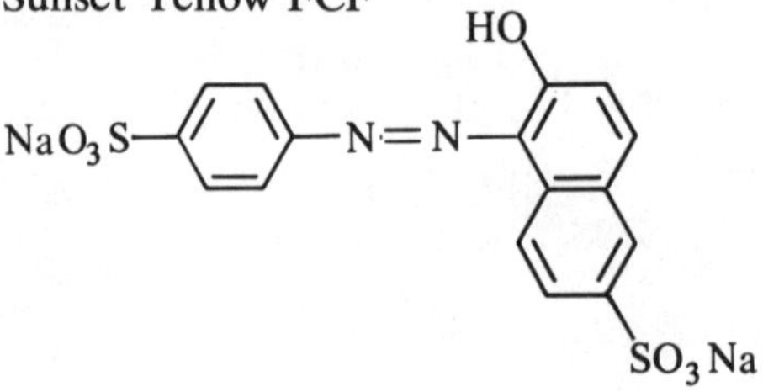

Patent Blue V

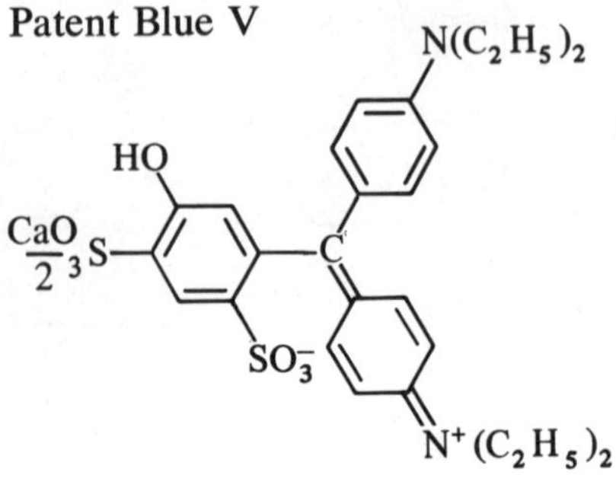

Violet BNP

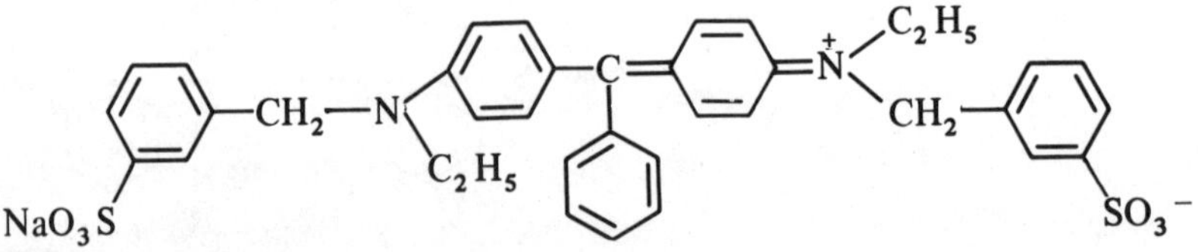

Some Dyestuff Food Colours in Current Use (*continued*)

Tartrazine

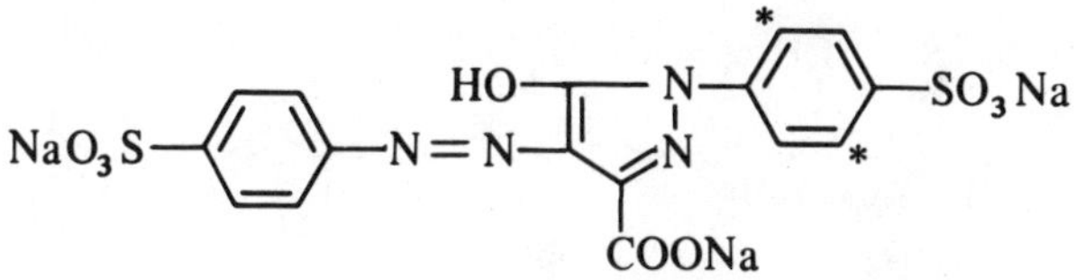

Note that Yellow 2G is basically similar to Tartrazine. It differs in having COONa replaced by CH_3 and by having dichloro substitution at points*.

Red 2G

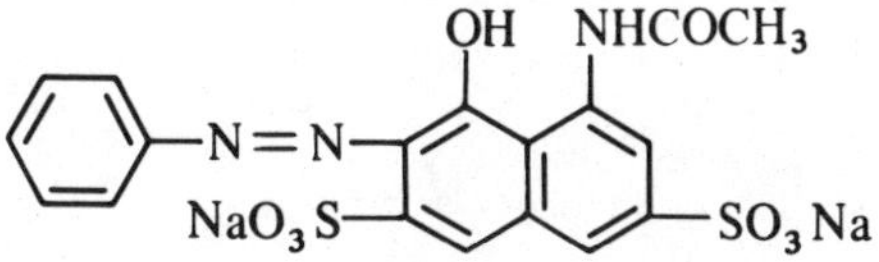

Note that in Red 10B NHCOCH₃ is replaced by NH₃.

So we find colours in one list and not in others, and colours admitted to the U.K. list and then rejected on second thoughts. By and large, the successive U.K. lists are illustrative of the rigorous pruning that has gone on over the years. The Japanese list is included to show not only its relative simplicity but also the mixture of common and uncommon colours. And of those that are common three are currently under a temporary ban. Two of the others have this in common with the preservatives, benzoic acid and 4-hydroxybenzoic acid[22,23] that they can promote an allergic response in sensitive people.

The switch away from dyestuffs has been facilitated by the isolation, identification, and synthesis of natural colouring substances, such as the carotenoids. Primary interest in synthesizing carotenoids[29] arose from a desire to produce β-carotene (provitamin A) as an extension of the synthetic work on vitamin A. In the event, its success also as a colour

NATURAL OR NATURE-IDENTICAL FOOD COLOURS

β-Carotene

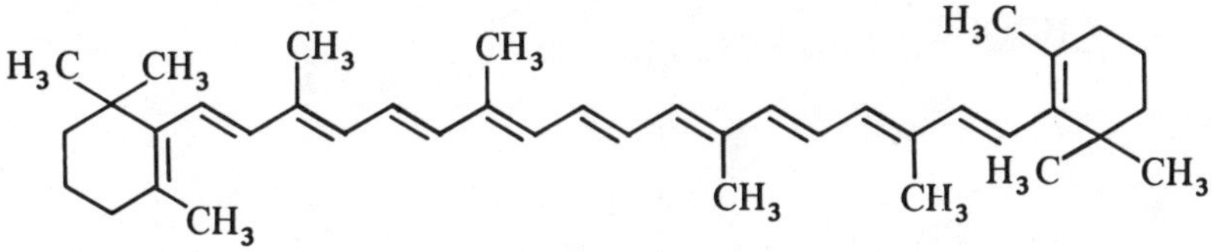

Natural or Nature-Identical Colours (*continued*)

β-apo-8'-carotenal

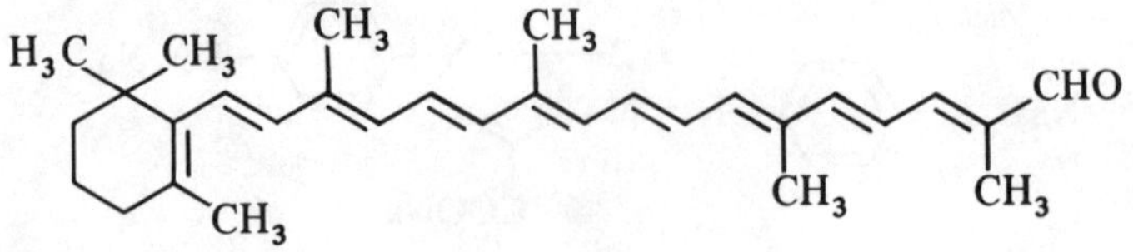

H₃C CH₃ CH₃ CH₃ CHO CH₃ CH₃

Ethyl β-apo-8'-carotenoate

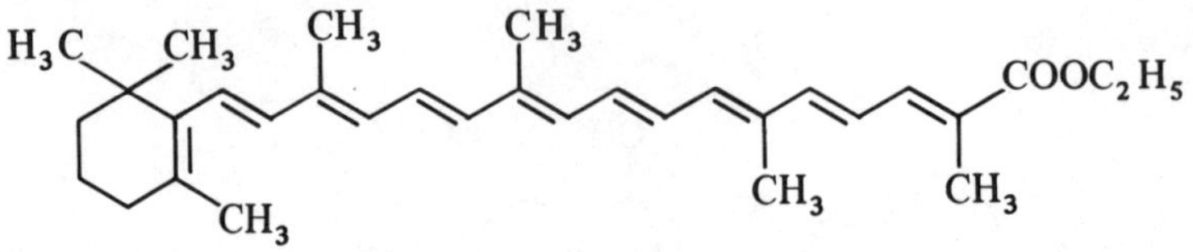

H₃C CH₃ CH₃ CH₃ COOC₂H₅ CH₃ CH₃

Canthaxanthin

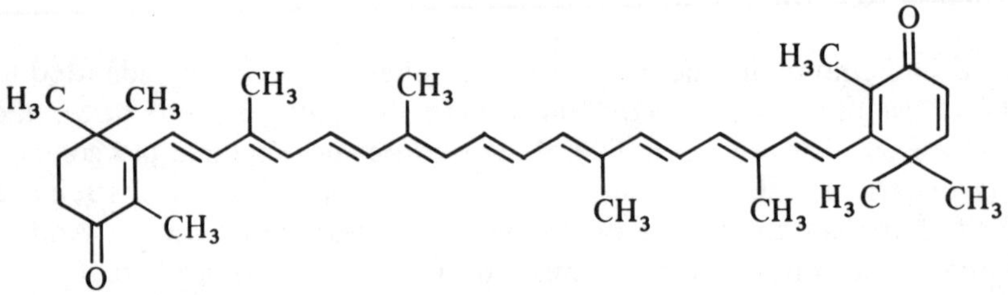

H₃C CH₃ CH₃ CH₃ H₃C O CH₃ CH₃ CH₃ H₃C CH₃ CH₃ O

Bixin

CH₃ CH₃ COOCH₃ HOOC CH₃ CH₃

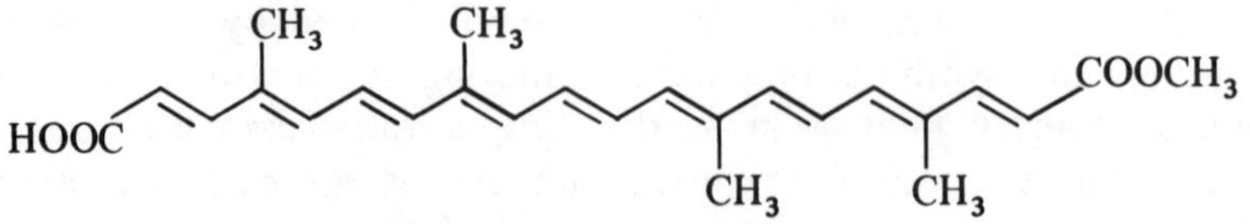

Crocetin (*ex* saffron)

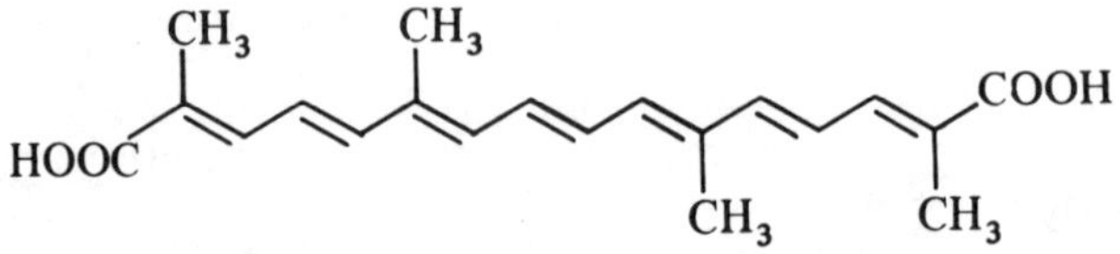

CH₃ CH₃ COOH HOOC CH₃ CH₃

Natural or Nature-Identical Colours (*continued*)

Beetroot Red

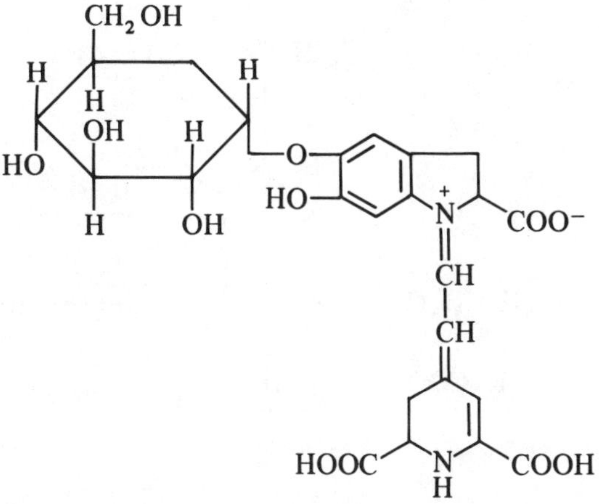

additive has led to the production of three other colour additives, β-apo-8′-carotenal, ethyl β-apo-8′-carotenoate, and canthaxanthin, the latter being a keto carotenoid. A number of these, as well as hydroxy carotenoids, occur naturally in fruits, berries, and leaves, etc., and extracts of these are also used. The carotenoid-like bixin, obtained from annatto seed, is also used.

Then there are the anthocyanins, produced by fruits and seeds, that provide colours ranging from red right through to blue; and extracts of beetroot, curcumin (turmeric), paprika, and saffron. There are, however, no nature-identical analogues available for these and supply is therefore limited. And finally we have chlorophyll, the green colouring material of plants. In nature it exists as a magnesium complex, but a deeper colour can be obtained by replacing magnesium with copper. It is interesting to note that, so far as nature is concerned, the colour of both chlorophyll and carotene is

Anthocyanins

R^2 is usually OH: R^1 and R^3 may H, OH, or CH_3, producing red, blue, or violet colours, the precise colour depending on pH.

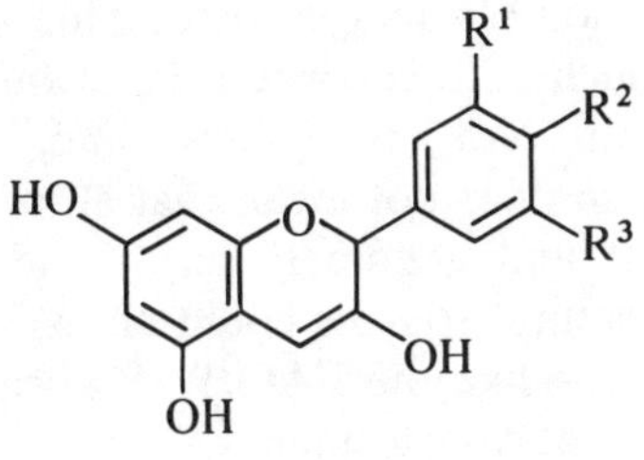

Nature or Nature-Identical Colours (*Continued*)

Chlorophyll a: in Chlorophyll b —CH$_2$ is replaced by CHO

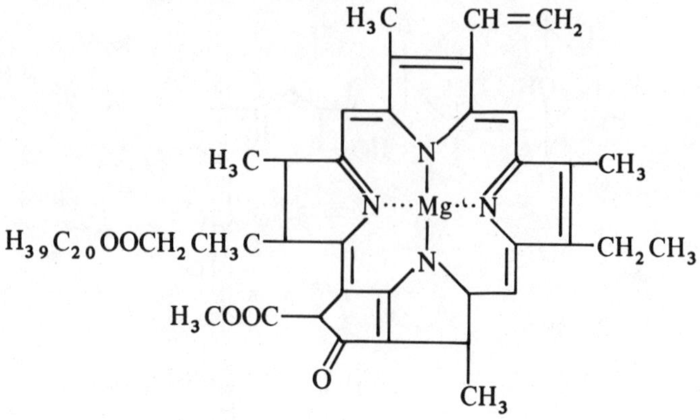

Curcumin

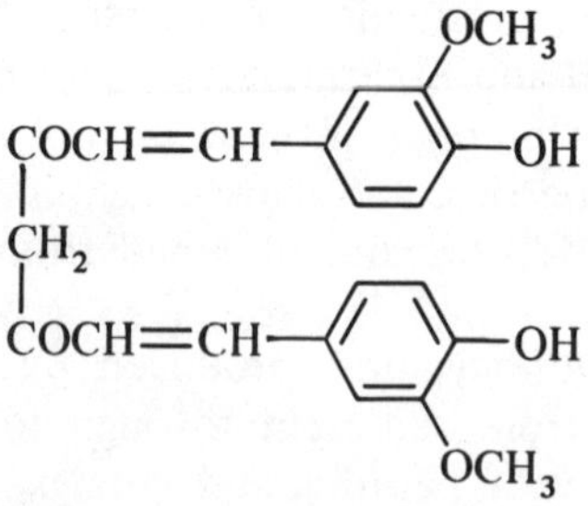

incidental. The sensitivity of a conjugated system to incident light has already been referred to. It can produce colour, but its significance here is to enable the two compounds to act in tandem, absorbing energy from the light source and using it to help photosynthesize plant growth. It just happens that the colours make the compounds useful food additives.

There is a long way to go before all food colour needs will be met from sources other than dyestuffs, but the movement away from dyestuffs will continue, even from those that carry no detectable hazard, for emotions die hard. Indeed the U.K. Food Additives and Contaminants Committee in its most recent communication[69] manages to combine sympathy with criticism when it states: 'That much of this concern is, in our opinion, based on an inadequate understanding of the facts and, in some cases, on misrepresentation of them does not mean that all of it is unjustified or that the concern is not real and genuinely felt.' And, while conceding that colours obtained from natural sources could be expected to be safe for use elsewhere, the Committee—like the FAO/WHO—calls for caution over the admissibility of nature-identical substances.

The U.K. communication is a review of the current situation concerning food colours. It has been concerned with identifying areas in which a revision of control seems advisable. It makes recommendations for future action. As a review, it is important not only for its survey of current U.K. practice, but for the underlying hope of tying that practice as closely as possible to EEC requirements; and for the detailed information—consistent with FAO/WHO wishes—that is provided on all colours, whether currently permitted or under consideration.

Readers with a passion for detail should consult the original communication. For the purposes of this book we need consider only certain aspects of it. First, discussions between the Scientific Committee for Food of the EEC and the relevant Committees of its member States have reached a point where it is possible in most cases to use EEC identification numbers for the colours and agreed ADIs (in mg/kg body weight). Second, the FACC have found it convenient to consider the use of colours relative to 19 classified groups of food commodities and to calculate for each group the amount of a given colour required. Third, the FACC have used their acceptability grading system to sort out the colours. There are 6 grades in all, but the colours to be considered here can be put into just three of them:

(A) Substances for which the available evidence suggests they are acceptable for use without qualification.

(B) Substances which are provisionally acceptable but require additional evidence of safety to be provided within 5 years.

(E) Substances on which there is insufficient evidence to express an opinion. One would have expected no substance in this grade to be recommended for even provisional use, and this in fact is the situation for all but one of the substances listed there. The one that does appear, Patent Blue V, is seemingly there because active toxicological investigation is in progress.

A fourth point to be noted is that the FACC have developed a basis for calculating what the average probable daily intake (in mg) of each food colour is likely to be in terms of what they call extreme diets, average diets, and children's diets. The Committee admits that a number of assumptions have had to be made in arriving at the figures, but the assumptions are applied consistently and the figures are comparable. For illustrative purposes, the figures for average diets, together with other interesting data, are given in Table 4.

Before dealing with the table, however, a number of other relevant details in the report must be noted.

1. Current regulations forbid the addition of colour to raw or un-processed meat, game, poultry, fish, fruit, vegetable, tea, coffee, coffee product, condensed or dried milk. Continuation of the ban relative to these is recommended.

2. Two dyestuffs, Chocolate Brown FB and Orange G are no longer in use in the U.K. and removal from the list of permitted dyestuffs is recommended.
3. It is not general practice in the U.K. to add colour to foods specially prepared for infants and young children. This is logical when one thinks of the reasons put forward for the addition of colour. The FACC consider that it would be advantageous to give this voluntary ban the force of an official regulation.
4. A quite unique situation with respect to caramel—normally a form of burnt sugar—which is used for both colouring and flavouring. In terms of the quantity used, caramel accounts for some 98% of all the colouring matter used in foods. However, there is a quite extraordinary multiplicity of methods for preparing caramel, resulting in something of the order of 100 different products. This makes it well-nigh impossible to characterize caramel for the purpose of regulation. It is proposed therefore, and work is in hand, to limit the various methods of preparation to, say, 6 and then to characterize and evaluate each of them.

Coming now to Table 4, the source reference for the information it contains is ref. 69 and it is important that whereas Table 3 dealt with permitted substances, or removals of permission, this one is concerned with recommendations for use.

It is to be noted that of the dyestuffs only four come into grade A acceptability, and it has to be added that one of them, Brilliant Blue FCF, is due for review at the end of 1980. Of those in grade B, which in general have 5 years of grace, four also are subject to review at the end of 1980. These are Brown FK (the kipper colour), Chocolate Brown HT, Red 2G, and Yellow 2G.

Possibly the most striking feature of the table—as the review itself points out—is that on an average body weight for an adult of 70 kg the probable daily intake for almost every colour for which data is available is well within the ADI for that colour. It should be evident to the reader, therefore, on this, the possibly most controversial of all additives, that not only is the matter not being treated superficially by the responsible authorities, but rather that there is more than a hint of extreme caution in approving any substance.

Flavours

Flavours are unique among food additives insofar as they have defeated all efforts to bring them under satisfactory statutory control: not that the public is thereby exposed to unnecessary hazard. Flavour ingredients overwhelm by the sheer weight of numbers. Any one natural flavour can be an amalgam of up to 50 component chemical substances, and a product

Table 4. Food Colours Recommended for Unconditional or Conditional Acceptance by the U.K. Food Additives and Contaminants Committee 1979. (For column Identification see footnote.) (Data used with permission of the Controller of Her Majesty's Stationary Office.)

I	II	III	IV	V	VI	VII	VIII
Brilliant Blue FCF		D	3	A	<0.005	2.5	175
Indigo Carmine	E132	D	10	A	0.03	5.0	350
Sunset Yellow FCF	E110	D	15	A	1.99	2.5	175
Tartrazine	E102	D	15	A	4.63	7.5	525
Amaranth	E123	D	13	B	1.44	0.75	52.5
Azorubine (Carmoisine)	E122	D	11	B	0.32	2.0	140
Brilliant Black PN	E151	D	4	B	0.01	0.75	52.5
Brown FK		D	5	B	0.21	0.05	3.5
Chocolate Brown HT		D	8	B	9.76	2.5	175
Erythrosine BS	E127	D	11	B	0.21	2.5	175
Green S	E142	D	13	B	0.08	5.0	350
Ponceau 4R	E124	D	12	B	0.88	0.15	10.5
Quinoline Yellow	E104	D	1	B	<0.005	0.5	35
Red 2G		D	7	B	0.31	0.1	7
Red 10B		D		B			
Yellow 2G		D	5	B	1.38	0.01	0.7
Riboflavin	E101	N	2	A	0.01	0.5	35
Riboflavin 5' (Na phosphate)		N		A			
Cochineal	E120	N	5	B	0.48		
Mg Chlorophyll	E140	N		A			
Cu Chlorophyll	E140	N		A			
Mg Chlorophyllin	E141	N		A			
Cu Chlorophyllin	E141	N		A			
Carbon Black	E153	N	2	A	0.09		
β-Carotene	E160(a)	N	9	A	0.23	5.0	350
Annatto	E160(b)	N	2	A	1.19	1.5	105
Bixin	E160(b)	N		A			
Norbixin	E160(b)	N		A			
Beetroot Red	E162	N		A			
Fe oxide and hydroxide	E172	N	1	A	0.11		
Ti oxide	E171	N	3	A	8.01		
Paprika spice		N		A			
Paprika *ex* spice		N		B			
Turmeric spice		N		A			
Turmeric *ex* spice		N		B			
Solvent-extracted annatto, bixin, and norbixin	E160(b)	N	2	B	1.19	1.5	105
Caramels		N	11	B			
Curcumin	E100			B			
Patent Blue V	E131	D	2	E	<0.005	2.5	175

I. Name of colour substance.
II. EEC code number.
III. Dyestuff (D) or non-dyestuff (N).
IV. Number of groups of food in which the colour is used, out of a total of 19 groups specified by the FACC.
V. Acceptability grade—A, B, or E.
VI. Average probable daily intake in mg by an adult.
VII. EEC recommended ADI in mg/kg body weight.
VIII. Calculated ADI in mg for a 70 kg adult.

38

formulator, aiming to incorporate a nicely rounded flavour, must count on the possibility that he may require a similar number of compounds to achieve his aim. He needs a large bank of substances from which to work.

The problem for those who have to determine whether individual substances are permissible or not is that, for many, there is only experience of a lack of complaint over many years use, and not toxicological proof of safety. But then, as we have already pointed out, this holds for many common sources of food.

A U.S. publication[30] provides many examples of flavouring materials in use, and of flavours or foods in which they have been used. But this compilation was produced in 1965, not to list permitted flavouring substances, but to establish the scale of use, as a guide to those contemplating legislative action. The difficulties are such that there has been little progress as yet.

Actually, the U.S. Food and Drugs Administration (FDA) had produced a list of 1124 flavour items that could be used in 1964, but the cyclamate scare of 1969 threw all additives under inquisitorial scrutiny and they are being slowly reassessed. The FAO/WHO Expert Committee on Food Additives is making its own equally slow assessment. By 1977[19] it had evaluated only 41 chemically identifiable flavour substances and established acceptable daily intakes (ADIs) for 35 of them. They also listed 9 flavour enhancers. Their findings are therefore of little practical help as yet.

The Japanese have simplified the problem by stating that natural materials can be used without restriction, but a nature-identical synthesis, or any other synthesized substance, must carry proof of safety. By this means they have produced a list of permitted substances of only 97 items,[27] but some of the items are multiple, e.g. aliphatic higher alcohols, and there is a repeated cautionary phrase, 'except harmful substances', which throws the onus on the user to establish a case. Most of the identifiable single substances in the Japanese list are to be found in the provisional U.K. list. There is, as yet, no kind of permitted list for the U.K. There, the Food Additives and Contaminants Committee has been proceeding with the benefit of hindsight, and with caution. It was aware of the confused situation in the U.S., and it had available a report produced in 1974 by the Council of Europe on Natural and Artificial Flavouring Substances. (How and why, of the whole span of additives, the Council came to be involved in this one class, is a matter for historians to unravel.) In the event the FACC's own report,[31] issued in 1976, provides an excellent review of earlier work and a workmanlike analysis of possible methods of dealing with flavours.

The Committee had material relating to 1585 flavour items and decided that they could be considered under six categories:

1. Natural flavouring substances which are, or are derived from, natural constituents of food, such as edible fruits or nuts. Eighty-three items were listed, their common and botanical names given, and the part of

the plant to be utilized named. One is reminded here of the observation in the previous section on food colours that it is permissible to remove a colouring substance from a food item and put it back at the same concentration; and one wonders again here what advantage is to be gained by removing a flavour from an already edible material and putting it into another one.

2. Natural substances consisting of, or derived from, vegetables, herbs, or spices, to be used in small quantities as additives to food, providing they are not used in quantities exceeding those occurring naturally in food. The same information was given as for category 1. Three hundred and eight-four items were listed, but there were limitations with respect to 73 of them because of specific toxic ingredients. This is interesting because many of them are present in plants that have a very long history of use. We will return to this point later.

3. Natural substances used at present, but whose sources are not at present widely consumed foodstuffs, herbs, or spices. One hundred and eleven items were listed. The committee saw no reason to ban them for the time being, but thought it advisable to have more evidence of their character and scale of usage.

4. Flavouring substances for which the evidence suggests possible toxicity and which should therefore be banned. There were only 13 items in this category and their sources are given here:

   Hepatica (*Anemone hepatica*)—herb
   Deadly Nightshade (*Atropa belladonna*)—whole plant
   White Bryony (*Bryonia dioica*)—roots
   Mexican Goosefoot (*Chenopodium ambrosioides*)—herb
   Lily of the Valley (*Convallaria majalis*)—whole plant
   Mezereon (*Daphne mezereum*)—whole plant
   Male Fern (*Dryopteris filix-mas*)—rhizomes
   (*Heliotropium europaeum*)—leaves
   Jamaica Dogswood (*Piscidia erythrina*)—roots
   Polypody (*Polypodium vulgare*)—rhizomes
   Pomegranate (*Punica granatum*)—roots
   Slippery elm (*Ulmus fulva*)—bark
   Squill (*Urginea scilla*)—bulb

5. Artificial and synthetic substances that the available evidence suggests are acceptable for addition to food, subject to stated limits of addition. Seven hundred and fifty-four items are listed. Both trivial and chemical names are given for each substance together with the formula. Furthermore the substances are classified on the basis of toxicological

evaluation as follows:

- a. No limit on addition except that determined by good manufacturing practice.
- b. Limit on technological grounds where toxicological level might be higher.
- c. Limit on both technological and toxicological grounds.

6. Artificial and synthetic substances which may be provisionally accepted for use in foods within set limits but on which some of the desirable toxicological data is lacking. Two hundred and thirty-four items were listed. They were classified as for the previous list except that class 1 named the kind of toxicological data that was missing for each item. They included one or more of the following:

- a. acute toxicity studies on selected species of animals;
- b. ninety day studies on sensitive species of animals;
- c. metabolic studies;
- d. proof of enzymatic hydrolysis;
- e. life-span study of one species of animal;
- f. tests for sensitization, i.e. allergic response.

Of the 1585 items considered, 597 were natural food substances and 988 were artificial or synthetic. In assessing the toxic risk the following factors were taken into consideration:

- i. levels of use;
- ii. whether used normally as food;
- iii. whether incorporated into staple items of the normal diet;
- iv. how the chemical structure compares with those of chemical compounds with known toxicological and biochemical behaviour;
- v. what self-limiting factors are present;
- vi. the contribution of a substance or any of its metabolites to the total dietary load;
- vii. possible losses during preparation, storage, or cooking of the food.

Thus recognizing that rigorous insistence on full toxicological testing on all submitted substances would be an impracticable task, it exercised judgement on what was required, and 234 items emerged as requiring further evaluations.

In a similar manner, it will be recognized that there are too many substances to permit any kind of comprehensive discussion here. One can only hope to convey a feeling of what has been involved and, to this end, it is a useful and illuminating exercise to consider those herbs and spices that are in common culinary use: if only to note that the chemical flavouring substances identified in them do not have the same immunity that has been accorded to the herbs and spices themselves through centuries of seemingly safe usage. In that sense it is illustrative also of the paradoxical situation that exists with regard to such flavouring materials, where experience has suggested safety while testing has disclosed a possible hazard.

First, what is the difference between herbs and spices? The Oxford Dictionary does not lead to an easy separation but, broadly, one tends to think of spices as originating in the Far East, and herbs in Europe, with something of an overlap in the Middle East. More often than not, herbs are perennial plants. The few plants that originated in America add a measure of complication to this simple mode of separation.

Known herbs and spices number many hundreds, and their primary use—and only use for most of them—is medicinal. No more than 50 find their way into culinary use. Selection and admixture of them for use is more an art than a science. As an art, the matter is of no great interest to us in the

TOXICANT SUBSTANCES IN HERBS/SPICES

β-Thujone

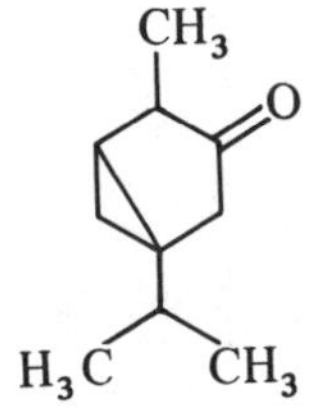

Coumarin

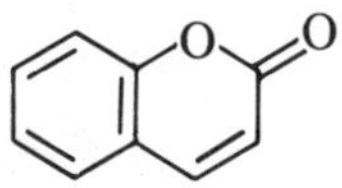

Caffeine

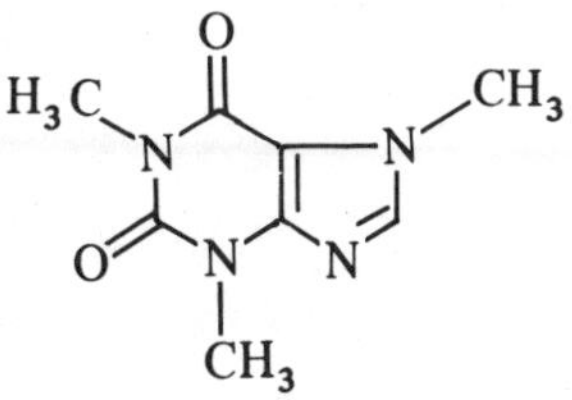

Pulegone

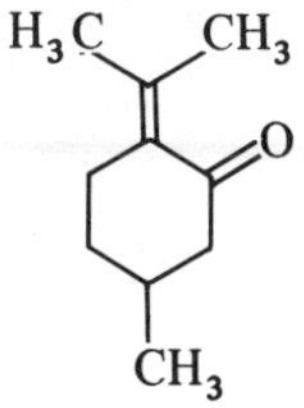

Hypericine

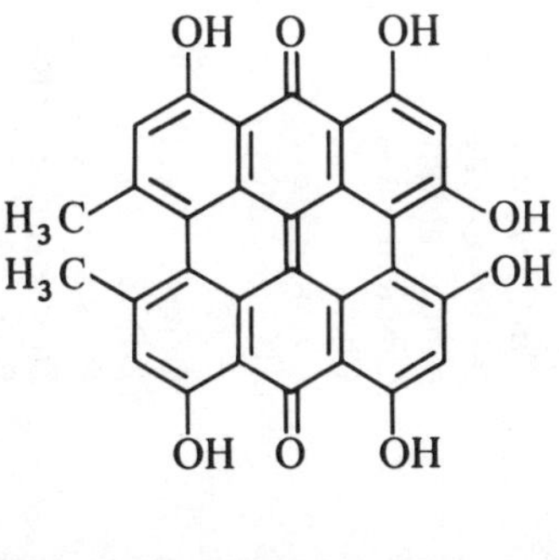

Safrole

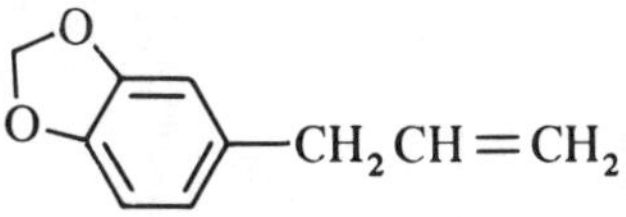

Methyl Nonyl Ketone

$$CH_3C(CH_2)_8CH_3$$

Table 5. Flavour Components Identified in Herbs and Spices

Component	Herb or spice	U.K. max. addition (mg/kg product)	FAO/WHO proposal (mg/kg body weight)
Allyl sulphide**	Garlic	1	
isoAmyl alcohol*	Peppermint	100	
Anethole*	Anise, fennel	340	0–1.25
Anisyl alcohol*	Vanilla	20	
Benzoic acid*	Anise lovage	250	
Benzyl alcohol*	Cloves	500	
Borneol*	Coriander, ginger, rosemary, thyme, nutmeg	10	
isoButyric acid*	Bay, parsley	no limit	
Cadinene***	Pepper	20	
Camphene**	Ginger	20	
d-Camphor**	Basil	10	
Carvacrol**	Oregano, lovage marjoram, savory	120	
Carveol**	Caraway	40	
4-p-Carvomenthenol**	Cardamon	50	
β-Caryophyllene**	Cloves, allspice, black pepper	50	
Cinnamaldehyde*	Cinnamon	700	
Cinnamic acid*	Vanilla	40	
Citral*	Ginger, pimento	50	
Cuminaldehyde*	Cumin	20	
p-Cymene*	Anise, coriander, cumin, mace, origanum	130	
Decanoic acid*	Anise	no limit	
2-Decanal*	Coriander	10	
Dihydrocarveol**	Black pepper	500	
Dipropyl disulphide*	Onion	5	
Estragole*	Anise, basil, pimento	40	

Compound	Source		
Eucalyptol*	Allspice, anise, basil, bay, etc.	20	
Eugenol*	Allspice, basil, bay, pimento	2000	0–5
isoEugenol*	Mace	30	
Farnesol*	Anise	5	
d-Fenchone*	Fennel	30	
Formic acid*	Mace	20	
Geraniol*	Bay, coriander, ginger, mace	30	
d-Limonene*	Anise, coriander	400	
Linalool*	Basil, coriander, ginger	40	0–0.25
Linalyl acetate*	Basil	10	0–0.25
Malic acid*	Vanilla	10,000	
Menthol*	Mints	1000	0–2
d-neoMenthol***	Japanese mint	150	
Menthone**	Peppermint	20	
Menthyl isovalerate*	Peppermint	50	
p-Methoxybenzaldehyde*	Fennel, anise, vanilla	50	
1-(p-Methoxyphenyl)-2-propanone***	Anise		
3-Methylbutyraldehyde***	Peppermint	30	
Methyl N-methylanthranilate*	Rue	5	
Myrcene**	Bay, pimento	no limit	
Myristic acid*	Lovage, mace	10	
Nonanal*	Ginger	5	
2-Nonanone*	Rue	10	
Octanal*	Lovage	no limit	
Octanoic acid*	Mace	50	
Perillyl alcohol**	Caraway	30	
Phenylacetic acid*	Japanese mint, black pepper	150	0–0.01
α-Pinene**	Anise, coriander, cumin, fennel, etc.		
β-Pinene**	Coriander, cumin, black pepper	100	
Piperidine*	Black pepper	5	
Piperine*	Black pepper	1	
α-Piperitone**	Japanese mint	20	

Table 5. (continued)

Component	Herb or spice	U.K. max. addition (mg/kg product)	FAO/WHO proposal (mg/kg body weight)
Piperonal*	Black pepper, vanilla	20	0–2.5
Propyl alcohol*	Onion	5	
p-isoPropylbenzyl alcohol*	Cumin, caraway	20	
α-Terpineol*	Cardamon, mace, marjoram, anise	40	
Terpinyl acetate*	Cardamon	20	
2-Undecanone*	Rue	5	
isoValeric acid*	Bay, parsley, peppermint, lovage	20	
Vanillin*	Vanilla	20,000	
Zingerone*	Ginger	20	0–10

*The compound has been placed in category 5 by the U.K. FACC.
**The compound is in category 6.
***The compound is not among those that have been considered.

present context. What is of interest is that although they have been used without challenge for centuries, present preoccupation with additives in general has brought them and their constituent chemical compounds under scrutiny, and has shown that some of the latter are only conditionally acceptable.[31] The following toxins have been identified in specific herbs, and limits for them in foods that contain the herbs, and in other foods, have been proposed according to the following list:

Thujone 10 mg/kg
Coumarin 5 mg/kg (alcoholic beverages 10 mg/l)
Caffeine 300 mg/kg
Pulegone 20 mg/kg
Hypericine 1 mg/kg
Methyl nonyl ketone 5 mg/kg
Safrole between 1 and 5 mg/l for alcoholic beverages;
    otherwise 1 mg/kg.

A list of flavour substances identified in herbs and spices is set out in Table 5. Of these only 10 appear in the FAO/WHO list[19] as having come under scrutiny. Information on natural herb or spice of each compound has come from reference 30.

Of the 66 substances listed, 63 are in the U.K. list, and 48 of them are to be found in category 5, that is, permitted for use but with upper limits on the level of addition. These limits, in fact, are of the same order as those to be found in category 6, and indeed to those with toxic hazards to be found in category 2 to which we referred earlier. What the Committee is saying in effect is that, if the usual cautious attitude is adopted here, then constituents of herbs and spices must be used with greater circumspection than has been historically used with herbs and spices *per se.*

Not unnaturally the U.K. authorities have now recommended that all herbs and spices, when used for flavouring, should be specifically controlled. This is logical, for it does not make sense that there should be control on component substances but not on the food items that contain them.

FLAVOUR COMPONENTS OF HERBS AND SPICES

Allyl sulphide

$(CH_2=CHCH_2)_2 S$

Anethole

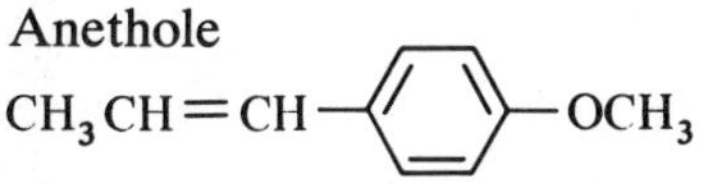

$CH_3 CH=CH-\langle\!\!\!\bigcirc\!\!\!\rangle-OCH_3$

Benzoic acid

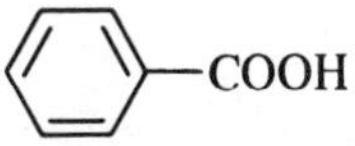

$\langle\!\!\!\bigcirc\!\!\!\rangle-COOH$

isoAmyl alcohol

$(CH_3)_2 CHCH_2 CH_2 OH$

Anisyl alcohol

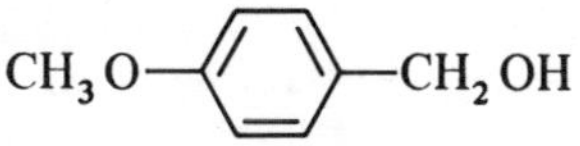

$CH_3 O-\langle\!\!\!\bigcirc\!\!\!\rangle-CH_2 OH$

Benzyl alcohol

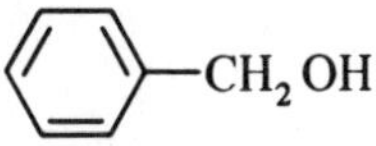

$\langle\!\!\!\bigcirc\!\!\!\rangle-CH_2 OH$

46

Flavour Components of Herbs and Spices (*continued*)

Borneol

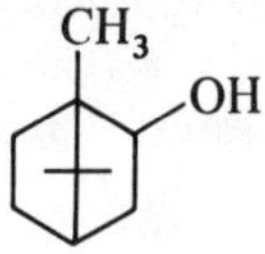

isoButyric acid

$(CH_3)_2 CHCOOH$

Cadinène

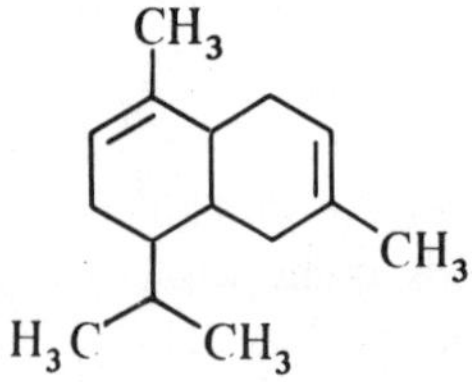

Camphene

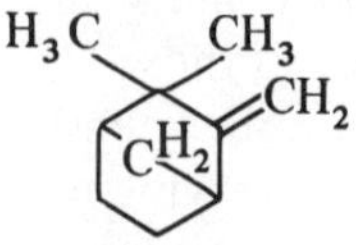

d-Camphor

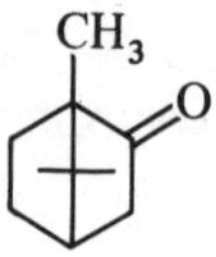

Carvacrol

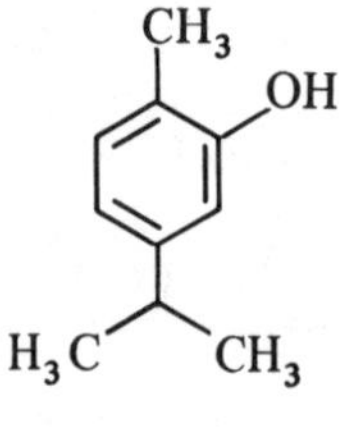

Carveol

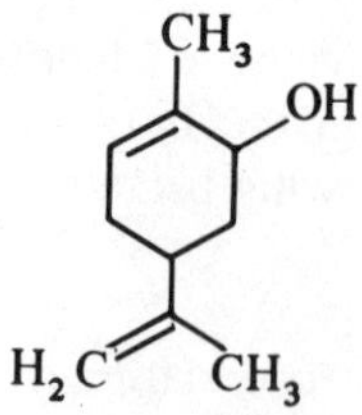

4-p-Carvomenthenol

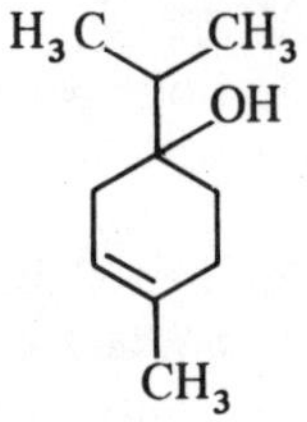

β-Caryophyllene

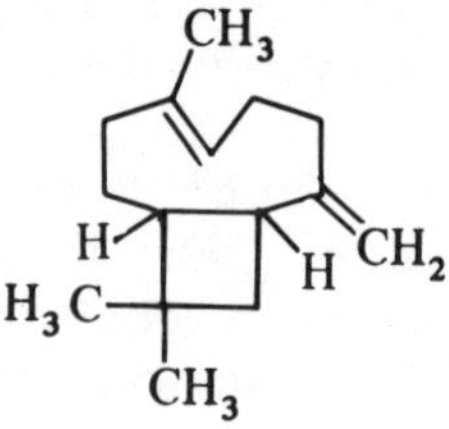

Cinnamaldehyde

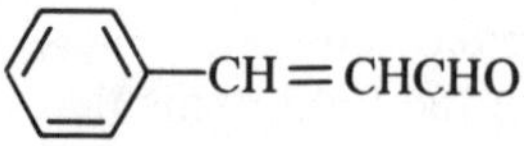

—CH=CHCHO

Cinnamic acid

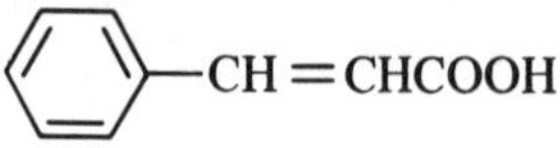

—CH=CHCOOH

Citral

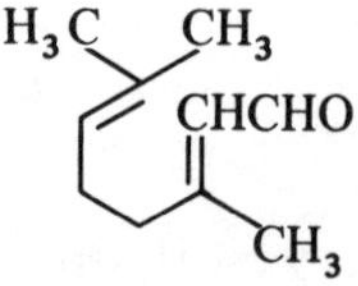

Cuminaldehyde

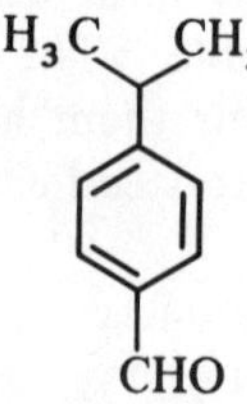

p-Cymene

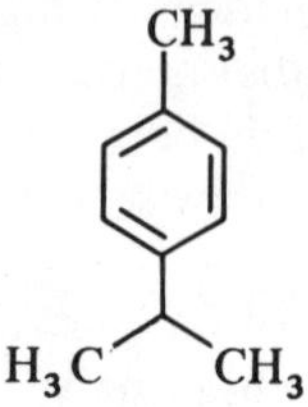

Decanoic acid

$CH_3 (CH_2)_8 COOH$

2-Decanal

$CH_3 (CH_2)_8 CHO$

Dihydrocarveol

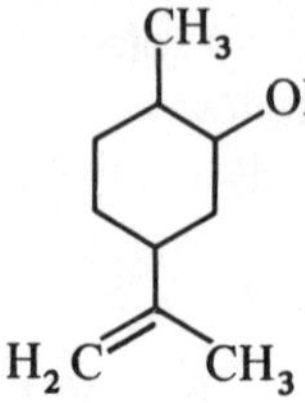

Dipropyl disulphide

$CH_3 (CH_2)_2 S—S(CH_2)_2 CH_3$

Estragole

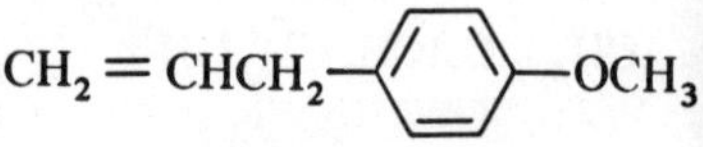

$CH_2 = CHCH_2-$ $-OCH_3$

Flavour Components of Herbs and Spices (*continued*)

Eucalyptol (Cineole)

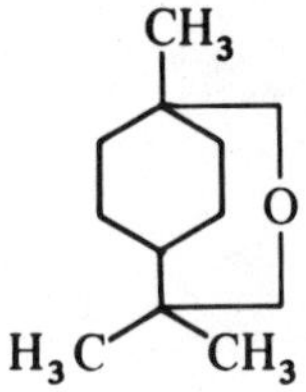

Geraniol

d-neoMenthol

$CH_2CH(CH_3)_2$

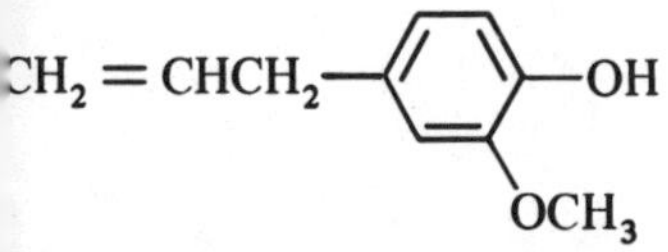

Eugenol

$CH_2=CHCH_2-$$-OH$, OCH_3

d-Limonene

Menthone

isoEugenol

$CH_3CH=CH-$$-OH$, OCH_3

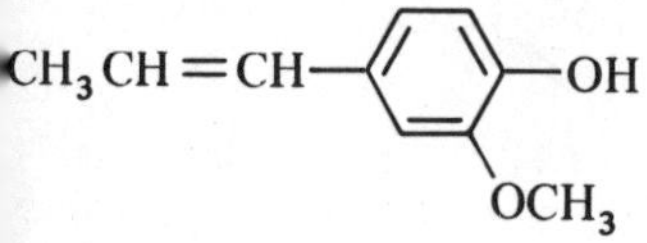

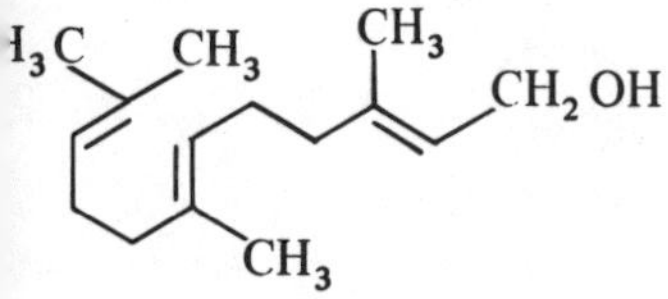

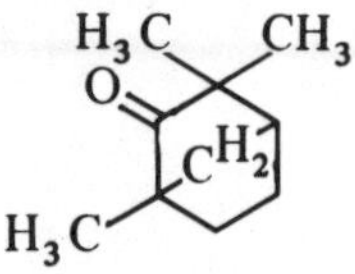

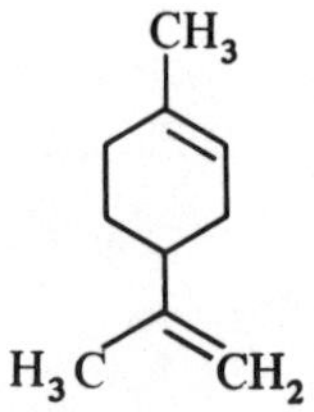

Linalool

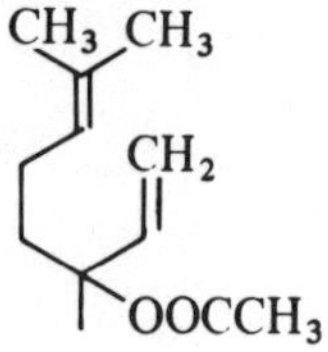

Menthyl isovalerate

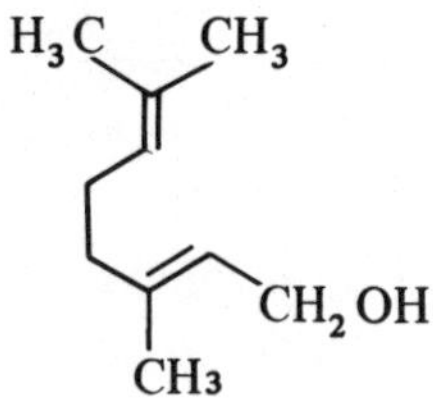

$OOCCH_2CH(CH_3)_2$

Farnesol

CH_2OH

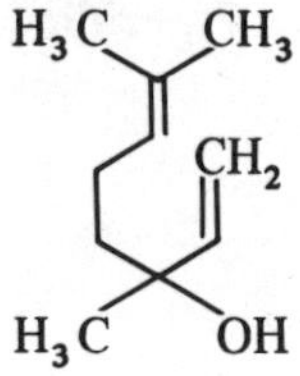

l-Malic acid

$HOCHCOOH$
$|$
CH_2COOH

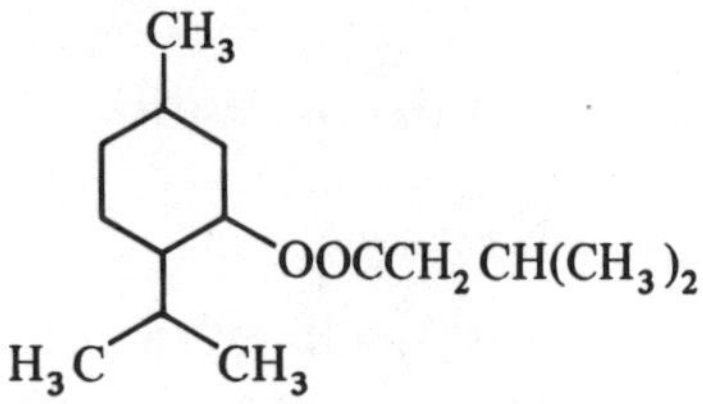

p-Methoxybenzaldehyde

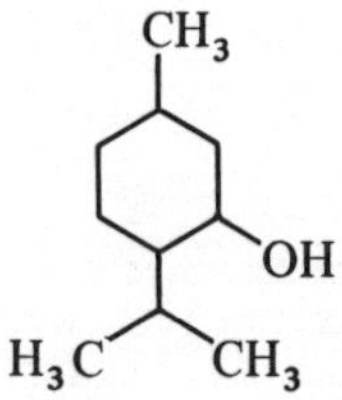

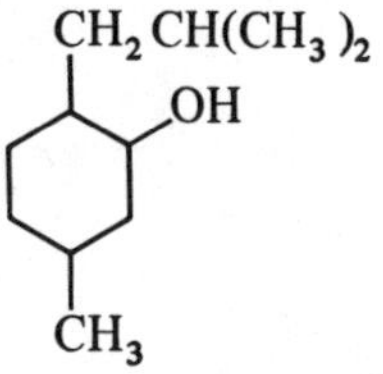

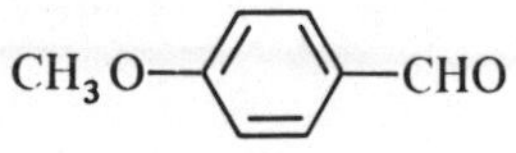

$CH_3O-$$-CHO$

d-Fenchone

Menthol

Formic acid

$HCOOH$

1-(p-Methoxyphenyl)-2-propanone

$CH_3O-$$-CH_2COCH_3$

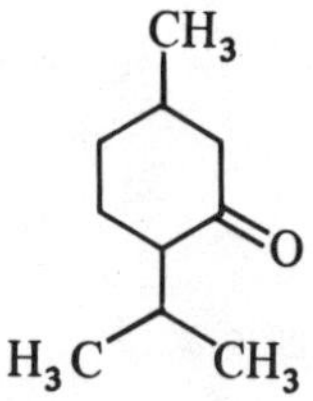

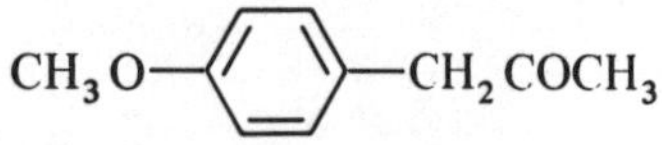

3-Methylbutyraldehyde

$(CH_3)_2CHCH_2CHO$

Linalyl acetate

$OOCCH_3$

48

Flavour Components of Herbs and Spices (*continued*)

Methyl *N*-methylanthranilate

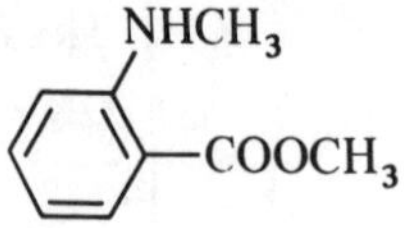

NHCH$_3$

—COOCH$_3$

Phenylacetic acid

—CH$_2$COOH

Myrcene

CH$_3$

CH$_2$

H$_3$C   CH$_3$

α-Pinene

CH$_3$

β-Pinene

CH$_2$

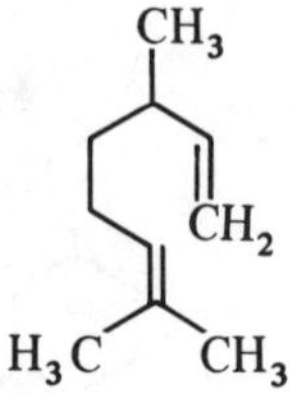

Myristic acid

CH$_3$(CH$_2$)$_{12}$COOH

Nonanal

CH$_3$(CH$_2$)$_7$CHO

Piperidine

H
N

2-Nonanone

CH$_3$(CH$_2$)$_6$COCH$_3$

Octanal

CH$_3$(CH$_2$)$_6$CHO

Piperine

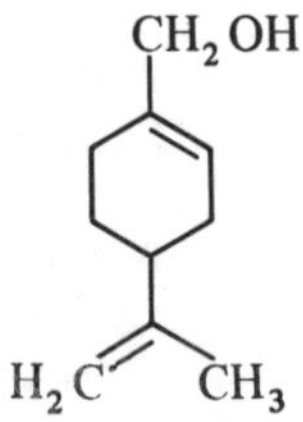

Octanoic acid

CH$_3$(CH$_2$)$_6$COOH

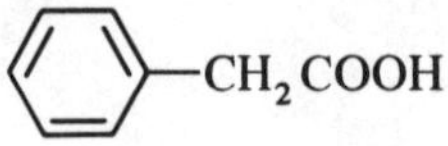

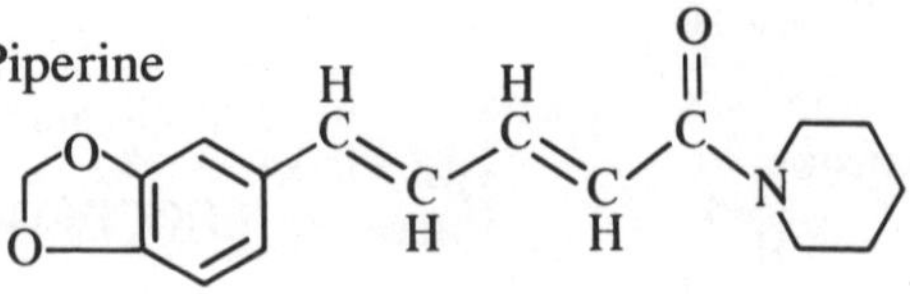

α-Piperitone

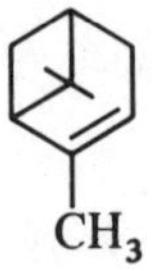

CH$_3$

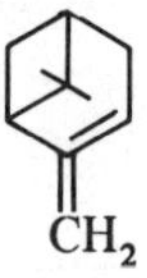

O

H$_3$C   CH$_3$

Perillyl alcohol

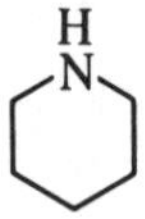

CH$_2$OH

H$_2$C   CH$_3$

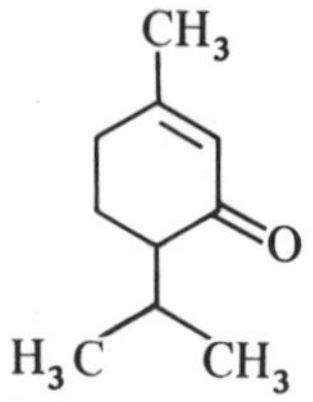

Flavour Components of Herbs and Spices (*continued*)

Piperonal

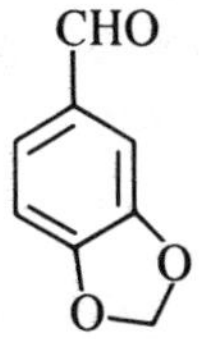

CHO

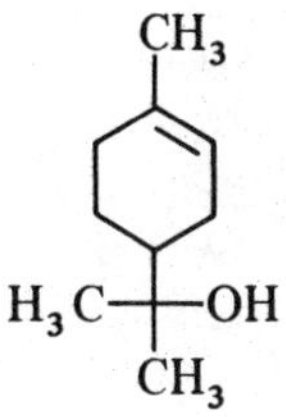

2-Undecanone

$$CH_3 CO(CH_2)_8 CH_3$$

isoValeric acid

$$(CH_3)_2 CHCH_2 COOH$$

Propyl alcohol

$$CH_3 CH_2 CH_2 OH$$

Vanillin

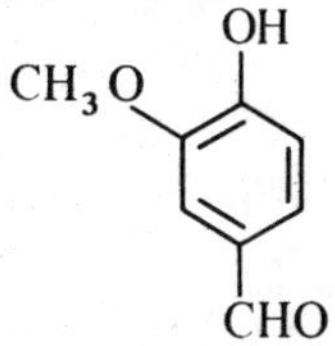

OH

$$CH_3 O$$

CHO

p-isoPropylbenzyl alcohol

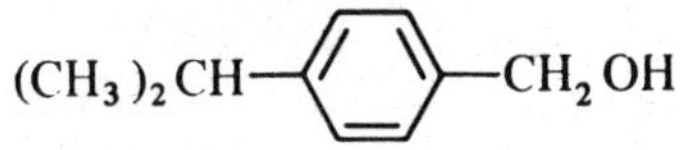

$$(CH_3)_2 CH—\!\!\langle\ \rangle\!\!—CH_2 OH$$

Zingerone

OH

$$CH_3 O$$

$$CH_2 CH_2 COCH_3$$

α-Terpineol

CH₃

$$H_3 C—\!\!|\!\!—OH$$
$$CH_3$$

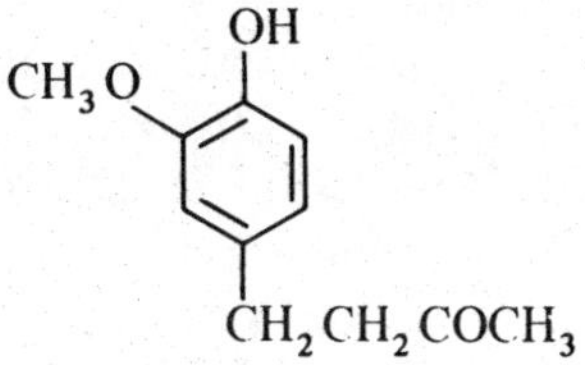

Sequestrants

In the section on antioxidants it was noted that certain metals, and particularly copper and iron, can act as pro-oxidant catalysts, and therefore need to be immobilized. Sequestrants are compounds that are added to do just this. Their composition is such as to have an affinity for a metal ion, and their molecular configuration is such as to provide a cage which prevents the metal ion becoming engaged in oxidative action. Most sequestrants are common substances, but the most effective is the synthetic compound ethylene diamine tetracetic acid (EDTA), which is used clinically in the treatment of metal poisoning.

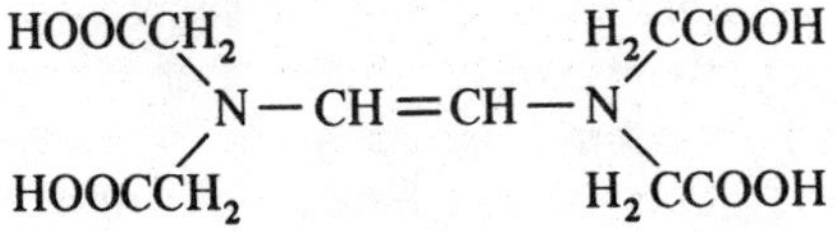

$$HOOCCH_2 \qquad\qquad H_2 CCOOH$$
$$N—CH=CH—N$$
$$HOOCCH_2 \qquad\qquad H_2 CCOOH$$

In food, in the form of the calcium salt, it has been found to work satisfactorily as a sequestrant without interfering with trace mineral metabolism, and the FAO/WHO list it[19] with an acceptable daily intake of up to 2.5 mg/kg body weight. However, the U.K. authorities prefer to limit its use[73] to canned fish and canned crustaceans, where it has been particularly effective in preventing the formation of struvite, needle-like crystals of ammonium magnesium phosphate.

The more commonly preferred sequestrants are phosphates and complex organic acids, and this understandable because both have an affinity for biological systems. Phosphates, for example play an important role in metabolic processes, and it is convenient that they should be used for the subordinate role of sequestrant.

By way of illustration it is to be noted that there are a number of phosphates which differ from each other in the ratio of H_2O to P_2O_5 and the power of sequestrant action depends on this ratio. Thus taking sodium orthophosphate, this will ionize to Na^{3+} and $(PO_4)^{3-}$. The negative ion can then pick up, say, a Cu^{2+} ion to form the complex ion $(CuPO_4)^-$ which will stay in solution. If sodium pyrophosphate had been used, this would have ionized to Na^{4+} and $(P_2O_7)^{4-}$, leading to the more strongly solubilized complex ion $(CuP_2O_7)^{2-}$.

Other permitted sequestrants are the tribasic citric acid, $CH_2COOH.HOCCOOH.CH_2COOH$, and its salts, and tartaric acid, $HOCHCOOH.HOCHCOOH$, and its salts. Here, it is likely that insoluble salts are formed and not soluble complexes. Finally, there is an amino acid in the U.K. list, yet curiously not in the FAO/WHO list although it is difficult to imagine any adverse affect since it is a common constituent of proteins. It is glycine, the simplest of all the amino acids, $CH_2(NH_2)COOH$, which will form a coordination complex with copper and other metal ions thus:

$$O=C-O^-_{\text{\\\\\\}} {}^{++}_{\text{\\\\\\}} {}^-O-C=O$$
$$H_2C-N^{\text{\\\\\\}}Cu^{\text{\\\\\\}}N-C$$
$$\quad\;\; H_2 \qquad\quad H_2\; H_2$$

Anticaking agents

Anticaking agents are anhydrous substances that can pick up moisture without themselves becoming wet and they are added to particulate products, such as dry mixes, to prevent the particles clumping together and so keep the product free flowing. They are either anhydrous salts that can be readily hydrated by binding the water, or substances that hold water by surface adhesion yet themselves remain free flowing. The latter are substances that either occur naturally in a near-crystalline but not completely crystalline state, or can be brought into the required state by suitable physical treatment. Many substances are polymorphic. That is to say, they occur in a number of crystalline states. These are states of low energy with strong interatomic bonding. This state is disturbed during a period of conversion from one crystalline order to another, and if the conversion can be arrested—as is always possible with a solid material—a material is obtained with unsatisfied bonding potential, otherwise known as surface activity. The phenomenon has many applications and drying is just one of them.

The FAO/WHO[19] list over 20 substances of both types, and they can be grouped as follows:

1. Salts of the long-chain fatty acids—myristic $(CH_3(CH_2)_{12}COOH)$, palmitic $(CH_3(CH_2)_{14}COOH)$, and stearic $(CH_3(CH_2)_{16}COOH)$. The following salts are permitted—aluminium, ammonium, calcium, potassium, and sodium.

2. Calcium phosphates.

3. Potassium and sodium ferrocyanide.

4. Magnesium oxide.

5. Salts of silicic acid—aluminium, magnesium, calcium, and a mixed calcium aluminium salt.

Compounds in groups 1,2, and 3 form hydrates. Those in groups 4 and 5 adsorb water, but magnesium oxide must be specially prepared to be in the right form to do so. In a sense, so must the silicates, but the mode of preparation—by precipitation of an hydrated silicate and subsequent drying—ensures that an active material is obtained.

It is strange to find ferrocyanide in this company, though the accepted daily intake is low, 0.025 mg/kg body weight. In any event, it is hard to conceive such a low permitted quantity having any significant effect.

The U.K. list[73] does not include it, and indeed keeps largely to adsorptive-type materials, though sodium pyrophosphate does appear. Two other phosphates, calcium phosphate and bone phosphate, are really adsorptive types. Bone phosphate is a peculiarly British product. It is made by calcining defatted bones and is basically calcium phosphate in a rather impure state, though the impurities, being of biological origin, are of no consequence. It is a relatively mild adsorbent and so is magnesium carbonate, also in the U.K. list. There are other magnesium compounds—the oxide, stearate, and trisilicate—together with silica, silicic acid, and calcium silicate. (Magnesium stearate is odd-man-out here, being hydrate forming.) Finally there are three rather more complex silicates—sodium aluminium silicate, sodium calcium aluminium silicate, and calcium aluminium silicate. They are similar in action but differ in alkalinity.

Although the U.K. list is shorter than the FAO/WHO list, it is still a little surprising that so many substances are needed, innocuous though they may all be. Differences in behaviour between the silicates, for example, are more subtle than significant.

Acids, Buffers, and Bases

An alternative title for this class of additives would be pH controllers, pH being a system of determining how acid or otherwise a material is. pH 7 represents a neutral situation. A value below that shows that the material is acid, and above it that it is alkaline. A buffer serves to keep the material at a predetermined pH. Acidic and basic states need no explanation. They can be achieved by the simple inclusion of a mineral acid or alkali. It is the buffered state, produced with the aid of weak organic acids, that requires some explanation. Let us consider it this way.

A weak acid is distinguished by the fact that it only partially dissociates in water to positive hydrogen ions, which are the basis of its pH value, and negative acid ions, and dissociation comes to a point of equilibrium. If the solution is titrated with a strong base, that is, one that dissociates fully, dissociated acid ions will be neutralized and, to restore the equilbrium, more weak acid molecules will dissociate. That is to say, the pH will be maintained. This is known as a buffering action, for the addition of the base would otherwise have raised the pH.

If we had started with a buffer salt there would have been an initial dissociation into basic and acidic ions, followed by interaction between the acidic ions and water to produce a similar associated/dissociated equilibrium.

Buffers are needed in the baking industry when carbon dioxide is used to make a batter porous, and in the soft-drinks industry to control the degree of acidity. The acids, or their salts, that are permitted call for no cautionary comment. The organic acids are:

Acetic acid	CH_3COOH	Lactic acid	$CH_3CH-COOH$
Succinic acid	$H_2C-COOH$		$\quad\quad\;\; \mid$
	$\quad\;\; \mid$		$\quad\quad\;\; OH$
	$H_2C-COOH$	Pyruvic acid	$CH_3C-COOH$
Tartaric acid	$HOCH-COOH$		$\quad\quad\; \parallel$
	$\quad\quad\; \mid$		$\quad\quad\; O$
	$HOCH-COOH$	Citric acid	$H_2C-COOH$
Malic acid	$HOHC-COOH$		$\quad\quad\; \mid$
	$\quad\quad\; \mid$		$HOOC-COH$
	$H_2C-COOH$		$\quad\quad\;\; \mid$
Fumaric acid	$HOOC-CH$		$H_2C-COOH$
	$\quad\quad\;\;\; \parallel$		
	$HC-COOH$		

Partial salts of the phosphoric acids—pyrophosphoric ($H_4P_2O_7$) and orthophosphoric (H_3PO_4)—as well as the free acids are also permitted. They all occur naturally in common foods.

Some fatty acids, both saturated and unsaturated, are permitted, though the lower members, butyric and caproic, are probably used as much for their flavour as for buffering potential. Pyruvic acid, mentioned above, though absent from the FAO/WHO list, also has a marked flavour.

There is little to say about permitted bases except to list them. Some are relatively weak—sodium sesquicarbonate, $Na_2CO_3NaHCO_3.2H_2O$, and ammonium and sodium bicarbonate. Some are strong—ammonium, potassium, and sodium hydroxides. And some lie in between—calcium and magnesium hydroxides, and the carbonates of all five.

It is to be noted that two of the weak organic acids, tartaric and citric, have already been listed as sequestrants, while the calcium salts of two sugar acids, gluconic acid and heptonic acid, which may also be used as buffers, appear later also as crisping agents. It is likely that the possible dual roles play a part in choice of one or other.

Humectants

Whereas anticaking agents are used to keep certain products dry, humectants are required to keep others moist, as for example, bread and cakes. Both kinds of additives do this by picking up water, but whereas anticaking agents immobilize it, humectants pass it on to the product to compensate for a natural drying out that would make the product unattractive. All humectants are hygroscopic and one of the commonest is glycerol, $CH_2OH.CHOH.CH_2OH$, but unfortunately, with a decline in the demand for soap—by which glycerol was produced during saponification of fat—as the popularity of non-soapy detergents grew, the availability of glycerol declined and alternatives had to be found.

One was propane-1,2-diol, $CH_3CHOH.CH_2OH$. Another was sorbitol, a sugar alcohol, $CH_2OH.HCOH.HOCH.HCOH.HCOH.CH_2OH$, which is also used as a sweetener. Other permitted substances, which can also serve as buffers are sodium and potassium lactate. But note: the FAO/WHO lists only the sodium salt as a buffer and humectant. It describes the potassium salt as an acid, preservative, and flavouring. Substances which serve a multiplicity of purposes must obviously be chosen to ensure that the possible ways that they act are compatible with the character of the product.

Firming and Crisping Agents

These are substances that preserve the texture of vegetable tissues and, by maintaining the water pressure inside them, keep them turgid. They do this by preventing a loss of water from the tissues. The FAO/WHO name 4 compounds: aluminium potassium sulphate, aluminium sulphate, calcium sulphate, and calcium hydroxide. The U.K.[73] name 8 compounds, one of which is common salt. Six are calcium compounds: the hydroxide, citrate, lactate, phosphate, gluconate, and heptonate. All have other additive roles and indeed, those not in the FAO/WHO list as firming or crisping agents appear there in one or other of the additional roles—buffer, preservative, emulsifier, etc. Thus insofar as safety, within specified limits, is really a property of a compound *per se* and not of its purpose in a food, absence from a particular list is not necessarily an indication of risk. Nevertheless, it should be noted that it would appear to be a preferred EEC practice that member countries identify each additive use where multiplicity occurs.

Sweeteners

Sweeteners are such a common constituent of foods that some may find it surprising that they are to be counted as a food additive. The most common sweetener is sugar, or more accurately sucrose since there are really a number of sugars. Few of the others have a marked sweetening effect. Some are poorly digested and liable to cause digestive upsets or other metabolic irregularities. And even common sugar—sucrose—is taboo for diabetics. This had led, in part, to an investigation into the basis of the response that we call sweetness, in the hope that it would lead to the discovery of new and preferable sweeteners, and in part to an empirical search.

There has been no real progress in the search for a theoretical basis for sweetness, and the most useful advance in the attempt to find alternative substances came—as so often happens in research—accidentally. In fact the substance, saccharin, had been noted, isolated, and identified as far back as 1880, and it was not the shortcoming of sucrose, but its shortage during the 1914–18 war, that brought saccharin into favour. As a compound having no calorific value, its advantage to diabetics, when that disease was identified, was immediately obvious; and also to obesity when that too came under scrutiny.

On the other hand, cyclamate did emerge from attempts to synthesize possible new sweeteners, and so did a dipeptide, which has been named aspartame. In the meantime there has been a continued search for natural sweeteners, particularly among tropical fruits known to be used by local people because they sweeten. But though much has been learnt about them, no practical application has yet emerged. One, thaumatin, is the most powerful sweetener yet discovered.[35] The fruit from which it comes has been used traditionally in Central and South West Africa to sweeten wines, maize bread, and sour fruit. It is proteinaceous in character and has been isolated. Unfortunately, the sweetness resides wholly in the way the protein chains fold in the native state, and anything that affects this folding, such as pH, temperature, or the breaking of links between peptide chains, destroys the sweetness. Much has yet to be done, therefore, before advantage can be taken of this remarkable substance.

In the meantime saccharin remains the most popular alternative to sugar though, for a time, cyclamate also came into wide use. Mixtures of the two, for example, were found to be technologically advantageous for addition to soft drinks. For, if sugar is given a sweetness rating of 1, the comparative

SWEETENERS

Sucrose

Saccharin

Sodium Cyclamate

Aspartame
L-Aspartyl-L-phenylalanine methyl ester

figure for saccharin was 300, and for cyclamate was 30. (That for thaumatin is of the order of thousands.) In other words, not only are saccharin and cyclamate non-calorific, but they are also much sweeter weight for weight.[33]

Faith in cyclamate, however, was shaken when laboratory reports from Canada brought it under suspicion as a possible carcinogen (see Chapter 4) and it was immediately banned in Canada, the U.S., and the U.K.: but not universally so: for, not only was the plan of the experiment in which the adverse result was obtained suspect, but the level at which the substance had been fed was grossly in excess of that at which it would normally be used.

The test, in fact used mixtures of saccharin and cyclamate in the proportions—but not the levels—normally present in soft drinks, and later tests with saccharin alone at the same level have produced a similar result to that on the mixture.[34] But saccharin has been used for at least 60 years without any kind of adverse reaction and a general ban is unlikely. In fact, only Canada has acted. What is really in question is the interpretation of the evidence and the judgement derived from it, and no doubt what happens in those countries which still permit it to be used will play a part in the ultimate judgement.

So the FAO/WHO still lists sodium and calcium cyclamate, though without an ADI. It also permits saccharin and its sodium and calcium salts—though not in infant foods—at a temporary ADI of up to 2.5 mg/kg body weight. There is also a limited permission for aspartame, which is the methyl ester of the dipeptide, L-aspartyl-L-phenylalanine, and has a sweetness rating of 180. Permission is limited because, like thaumatin, it is sensitive to pH and temperature and the effects of changes due to these have not yet been fully examined.

Meanwhile, there has been a new look at monosaccharide sweeteners, and sorbitol is now used in confectionery, or mannitol if the confectionery is calorie reducing, and xylitol in chewing gum, although the safety-in-use of xylitol is now suspect.

Enzymes

Enzymes have excited the interest of scientists for many years. It did not take so long to find out what they could do, but it took much longer to find out what they were. Even as late as 1950 all that could be claimed was that the few enzymes that had been identified all had a proteinaceous character. We now know that they comprise one class of proteins and have no distinctive features that would mark them chemically from other kinds of proteins. So, in order to understand enzymes, we must first think of them as proteins, before we consider the behaviour that distinguishes them as enzymes.

Proteins are composed of amino acids, for which the general formula is

$$R-CH-COOH$$
$$|$$
$$NH_2$$

Thus we have within the molecule a basic group, NH_2, capable of coupling with an acidic group, an acidic group, COOH, similarly capable of coupling with a basic group, with the elimination of water in each case. This is, in fact, the way in which the first stage, and sometimes the only stage, of protein synthesis takes place.

$$R^1-CH-COOH + R^2-CH-COOH \longrightarrow R^1-CH-COOH + H_2O$$
$$\qquad NH_2 \qquad\qquad NH_2 \qquad\qquad\qquad NH$$
$$\qquad\qquad\qquad\qquad\qquad\qquad\qquad R^2-CH-C=O$$
$$\qquad\qquad\qquad\qquad\qquad\qquad\qquad\qquad NH_2$$

In this way a polymeric chain will build up which we will set out thus:

$$\ldots -NH-CH-C-NH-CH-C-NH-CH-C-NH-CH-COOH$$
$$\qquad\quad R^4 \qquad\qquad R^3 \qquad\qquad R^2 \qquad\qquad R^1$$

If one tried to build this with models one would find that the polymer would not actually stretch out in a straight line but form into a spiral. We call the complete spiral chain a peptide and the size of it is predetermined and depends on the kind of protein it is a part of.

The R groups are important. There are 20 different amino acids involved in protein synthesis and each is distinguished by the R group. Some are paraffinic, that is, they contain only carbon and hydrogen in characteristic paraffinic formations. Others have OH, or NH_2, or COOH, or S in the side grouping. Thus the side groups provide a range of affinities which can lead on occasion to chemical bonding, to electrostatic attraction, or to what is known as hydrogen bonding when, for example, $=O$ and H–O– lie close enough to each other. All this depends on how adjacent peptide chains lie relative to each other and how they fold. And this in turn is predetermined by the order in which selected amino acids are used to build up a specific peptide.

So we find some proteins constructed to act structurally as in muscle, with the power of extension and contraction. And others to have a physiological purpose, such as globin, which can fold in a precise manner to form a cage that will hold an iron-containing haem group. The precision of this is underlined by the incidence of sickle cell anaemia, named after the shape of the red blood cell in patients who suffer from the disease. Globin contains some 300 amino acids, yet the replacement of just one, glutamic acid, in a specific site, by valine is sufficient to upset the normal behaviour of haemoglobin.

The biggest of all the groups of proteins is that of the enzymes and this is not surprising for they are the key to all metabolic processes that go on within a living organism of any kind, and each process requires its own set of enzymes. Some of those processes are of interest to food manufacturers, and the enzymes involved then serve as food additives.[36]

A simple comparison between enzymes and other proteins would be to say that whereas the latter were the consequence of metabolic activity within the organism, the latter were not only that but also operators of metabolic activity. To repeat what I have written elsewhere. 'Living organisms are engaged for the most part in a furious activity in which proteins are engaged both actively and passively—building, transforming, and destroying—and being built, transformed, and destroyed. Most of them exist in a state of permanent impermanence.' Those that are enzymes achieve their character by the selection and arrangement of R groups along the various peptide chains so that, when the protein folds, it takes up a shape that aligns specific intramolecular forces. Each enzyme, in fact, is shaped for a specific job, not only in attacking, say, a lipid or a carbohydrate or another protein, but just where within the molecule it attacks.

It has been aptly described as a lock and key effect insofar as, to the best of our knowledge, there must be a fit between the enzyme molecule and that to be split: a fit however that must produce a strain, to allow intermolecular forces to break the chemical bond. Because they enable such changes to take place, they were known, in the days before their proteinaceous character was recognized, as organic catalysts; but perhaps they are better described as the worker bees of the biological system, carrying out predestined roles that involve construction or demolition of biological material. They are identified by what they interact with: lipases, carbohydrases, proteases, oxidases, reductases, and so on. The precise structure of quite a number of enzymes has now been worked out and the lock and key theory substantiated.

The digestive system may be considered one of finely controlled degradation of food by enzymes, control being provided by pH, temperature, and concentration of the enzyme. A number of uses of enzymes in the food industry stem from knowledge of the digestive system. Other uses come from acute observation by our forebears: observation that predates knowledge that enzymes were involved. The latter include the making of leavened bread, of cheese, and of yoghourt. And it is to be noted that the modern process of meat tenderizing had its roots in methods used by primitive tribes in Central America, who were observed to rub the juice of papaya leaves into meat, or to cut the meat into small pieces and wrap them in papaya leaves before cooking.

Food scientists now know, and make use of the fact, that an enzyme, papain, was attacking the crosslinks that form with age between muscle fibres and within a mass of collagen (ultimately to form gristle). Actually papain is more effective with muscle than with collagen; but two other enzymes have since been identified, bromelain (from pineapples) and ficin (from figs), that work better with collagen. Anyone who has attempted to masticate mutton from a three or four year old sheep, or one of the cheaper cuts of beef, will readily recognize the need for tenderizing; for such meat, though good in a nutritional sense, is otherwise unattractive and almost indigestible. In an era when the world's protein resources present a serious problem, it is important to maximize utilization of what is available.

For the same reason, meat scraps and fish waste from the processing industries, though highly unattractive as food to a sophisticated society, need not be discarded, for their nutritional value is high, and indeed is not held to be unattractive by more primitive societies. However, all tastes can be satisfied by reducing them to hydrolysates by means of the digestive enzymes, pepsin and trypsin. These break down the muscle proteins to smaller peptidic units that are small enough to go into colloidal solution. As such, they have a number of applications in modern food technology, and they have a special application to people who have undergone a period of starvation, and who can thus be fed specially balanced hydrolysates in order not to overtax their digestive system when breaking their enforced fast.

All the enzymes mentioned above are proteases, that is, enzymes that attack proteins in one way or another, and there is one more to be mentioned, rennin, which is used in cheesemaking. The traditional source is a crude concentrate, rennet, prepared from the stomachs of calves. But not only does demand exceed supply from this source today, but there are also ethnic and religious scruples to be taken into account. So alternative sources have been sought and a number have been found: all, somewhat surprisingly, microbial—*Bacillus cereus, Endothia paraciticus, Irpex lacteus, Mucor michei,* and *Mucor pusillus.* Control of such sources is discussed below.

The action of rennin is to reduce a 'water-soluble' milk protein, caseinogen, to casein, which then interacts with calcium present in the milk to form a cheese curd.

A number of non-protease enzymes are also of interest, and of these we will first consider glucose oxidase, which is used to prevent what is known as the Maillard—or browning—reaction between the aldehydic group of sugars and amino groups of proteins. Not that the reaction is always unwanted, for it helps to produce the colour and flavour of such products as bread, cakes, breakfast cereals, and roast meat. But it is not wanted in dried eggs, dried meat, and dehydrated potatoes.

This enzyme will also remove oxygen and has been used for this purpose in a number of processes: stabilizing citrus-juice-based soft drinks; co-stabilizing vitamins B_{12} and C in aqueous preparations; preventing rancidity (i.e. acting as an antioxidant) in oil/water emulsions, or oxidation of beer, or vinegarization of wine, or the browning of fresh fruit. The enzyme is isolated from the mould, *Aspergillus niger,* and this remains the principal source.

Next there is catalase, a peroxidase, which has found use both in the dairy industry and in the pasteurization of eggs. It acts on hydrogen peroxide to release oxygen and produce water. There is, in fact, a coupled reaction in which one molecule of peroxide is oxidized and another reduced:

$$H_2O_2 \longrightarrow H_2 + O_2$$

$$H_2O_2 + H_2 \longrightarrow 2 H_2O$$

In the dairy industry the enzyme is used to remove residual peroxides from milk that is to be used for cheesemaking, and also to stabilize and enhance the action of milk-souring cultures. The principal sources of the enzyme are *Aspergillus niger* and *Micrococcus lysodeikticus*. It is present in bovine liver but this does not provide a commercial source.

Finally there are the carbohydrases, and amylase in particular. Carbohydrases attack polysaccharide linkages and produce smaller and more easily digested sugar units. They are used for this purpose in the baking industry, and also for making 'modified starches', which can act as emulsifier stabilizers. Again the sources are microbial: *Arthrobacter, Aspergillus niger, Aspergillus crysae, Saccharomyces* spp., *Bacillus subtilis*.

The FAO/WHO Expert Committee on Food Additives (Chapter 5), in considering the safety aspects of enzyme preparations proposed for use in food processing,[37] has noted:

> 'Only in exceptional cases are these enzymes used as crystallised pure substances. From the safety point of view the presence of potentially harmful contaminants and byproducts is of concern. The nature and level of these substances may vary according to the sources selected for the preparation of the enzyme, the culture and the extraction procedures. Moreover, when microorganisms are used for the production of enzymes, mutations might occur that could lead to the emergence of new, potentially toxic products. The Committee felt that chemical and microbiological specifications and the biological control of strains of microorganisms used to produce these food enzymes are of the utmost importance in assuring the safety of these materials.' 'The increasing use of immobilised enzymes calls for the evaluation of the immobilising substance as well as the immobilising techniques.'

Thus the Committee laid down clear guidelines for dealing with enzymes. They further identified five classes of enzymes as follows:

1. Enzymes obtained from edible tissues of animals commonly used as foods. These were to be regarded as foods and consequently considered acceptable if satisfactory chemical and microbiological specifications could be established.

2. Enzymes derived from plants, more specifically, edible parts therefrom. These are also to be regarded as foods and consequently considered acceptable if satisfactory chemical and microbiological specifications can be established.

3. Enzymes derived from microorganisms that are traditionally accepted as constituents of food, or are normally used in the preparation of foods. The same comments hold as for classes 1 and 2.

4. Enzymes derived from non-pathogenic organisms commonly found as contaminants in food. These materials are not to be considered as foods. The Committee considers it necessary to establish chemical and microbiological specifications, and to conduct short-term toxicity experiments to ensure the absence of toxicity. Each preparation of the enzyme must be evaluated individually and an ADI must be established.

5. Enzymes derived from microorganisms that are less well known. These materials require chemical and microbiological specifications and more extensive toxicological studies, including a long-term study with a rodent species.

Preparations of all the enzymes named earlier have been considered by the Expert Committee.[38] Most of them have been found acceptable in defined conditions of use, but decision has been postponed on nine of them, not because there is evidence of hazard, but because adequate proof of safety is still lacking. The nine are ficin; carbohydrase, protease, and lipase ex *Aspergillus orysae spp.*; rennet ex *Irpex lacteus*; catalase ex *Penicillium amagasakiense*; and carbohydrase ex *Arthrobacter*.

The U.K. authorities are currently still considering the status of enzyme preparations. Meanwhile the FAO/WHO recommendations serve as guidelines, and the 1955 Food and Drugs Act as an overall safeguard.

Nutritive Additives

An adequate diet requires not only a proper quantity and balance of proteins, fats, and carbohydrates, and of essential amino acids within the protein moiety, but also that the main constituents should be acting as carriers for certain important though minor constituents of the diet—vitamins, trace elements, and minerals. To help ensure this, it has become common practice, when normal dietary articles of food do not, for one reason or other, between them provide sufficient of the minor constituents, to select a suitable food to act as vehicle for a constituent in deficiency. Thus margarine is fortified with vitamins A and D, and white flour with calcium, iron, and the vitamins, thiamin and nicotinic acid. And baby foods must contain such quantities of nutrients that, when fed as prescribed, they provide the recommended amounts, set out in Tables 1 & 2 in Chapter 1.

Vitamins

Most readers will know that many vitamins have now been synthesized, and they may know that the synthesized version is often used preferentially because its purity can be guaranteed. The food processor then knows exactly what he is working with. They may also be aware that there are those who claim a 'natural' vitamin to be superior to the synthetic copy. This is a nonsense, of course. All vitamins are identifiable chemical substances, which achieve their effect because of some specific feature in their chemical constitution. There is nothing mystical about the matter. What is mystical is that those which originate in plants or bacteria, with specific roles to play there, play other vital roles in the human organism.

The name vitamin has been given to a heterogeneous group of substances that have only two things in common: they are required in only trace quantities in the diet, and they are essential to metabolic processes within the body. Chemically they bear little or no relationship to one another. Many require a trace element to activate them. One—vitamin B_{12}—incorporates the element. Nowadays, therefore, vitamins and trace elements are often grouped together as micronutrients.[42]

Vitamin A is a complex alcohol which is required for growth, good vision, controlled tissue growth, and reproductive ability: a strange amalgam of properties of which the part it plays in vision is the only role reasonably well understood; though there is evidence that suggests that in tissue growth it intervenes to prevent soft tissue, and round the eyes in particular, hardening to a kind of keratin. The main source of the vitamin today is via synthesis, but it is available in liver oils. It is not available from plant sources though some writers claim erroneously that it is. What is available is its precursor, β-carotene, and this is absorbed by the body only if there is sufficient fat in the diet to facilitate this. Lack of fat has led to deficiency disease on occasion in African tribes that have plenty of carotene in their diet. Theoretically, one molecule of carotene would yield two of vitamin A by a symmetrical split, but the body is not very efficient at this and, even under optimum conditions, produces only some 60% of the theoretical yield. Furthermore, if there is adequate vitamin A in the diet, the body does not bother to split it at all, but rejects the carotene. The cow does better, getting its carotene from the grass it eats, and having a rumen to do the splitting. From there the vitamin passes partly to the milk, and hence to butter made from it, and partly to the cow's liver for its own use. For this reason, butter made from spring milkings, when the pasture is most lush, is richer nutritionally than any other.

Vitamin A is added to margarine to match the average content of butter, and in Eastern countries to vanaspati to match ghee.

Vitamin D is a particular kind of sterol, of which there is no shortage for man only if he happens to live in hot sunny climates. In temperate and less sunny places he had formerly to rely on fish or animal sources, though now a substance with the properties of vitamin D is produced from a plant sterol. Why certain fish and animals can produce the vitamin in climatic conditions that do not suit humans is a mystery. The vitamin is stored in the liver and it is used to help synthesize a carrier protein that transports calcium from the gut to a site of bone formation. A gross shortage leads to rickets in the young and osteomalacia in the elderly. In a sense, Nature has slipped up so far as humans are concerned, for the body is quite capable of producing its own supplies, given enough sunlight; for the last stage of biosynthesis is in the skin (that's one reason why furry animals lick their fur). But there is not sufficient sunlight in Britain for photosynthesis to be effective, and that is why immigrant Pakistanis, keeping to their native diet, run a risk of vitamin D deficiency. In Britain the vitamin is added to margarine at a considerably higher level than it occurs in butter to ensure that children have an adequate supply.

Vitamin E is a tocopherol that has already been mentioned as an antioxidant. It occurs naturally only in seed oils and so must be present in the diet. Its main biological role is also as an antioxidant, protecting the unsaturated essential fatty acid, arachidonic acid, in cell membranes. All membranes have a lipid/protein interface and the efficiency of the vitamin action is dependent on the presence in the proteinaceous phase of the trace element selenium, or rather of a seleno-enzyme, that is, an enzyme that needs to contain selenium in order to function properly. It has been postulated that the vitamin, in protecting the lipid, helps to maintain an environment in which the seleno-enzyme can function. Disorders due to a shortage of either the vitamin or selenium have been observed in premature babies, in patients suffering from intestinal malabsorption or obstructive jaundice, or from a rare congenital disorder that leads to a shortage of the lipoprotein that acts as a carrier for the vitamin in the blood stream.

Vitamin K belongs to a group of substances known as quinones and it takes part, in the liver, in the synthesis of prothrombin, a protein that causes the blood to coagulate. There are two active forms. One is present in green vegetable foodstuffs, the other is produced in the intestines as a result of bacterial activity there. However, absorption from the gut requires the presence of bile salts, and these may be unduly restricted in cases of obstructive jaundice, with a risk of excessive bleeding during surgical treatment. Also, newly born infants lack the necessary bacterial flora and rely on the mother's milk, or other source, for initial supplies.

The formulae given for the above four vitamins show them to be very different chemically, but they have this in common, that they are all

NUTRITIVE ADDITIVES

Vitamins

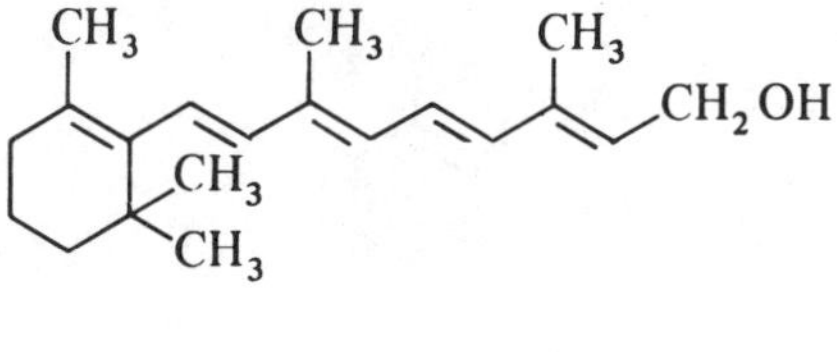

Vitamin D (cholecalciferol)

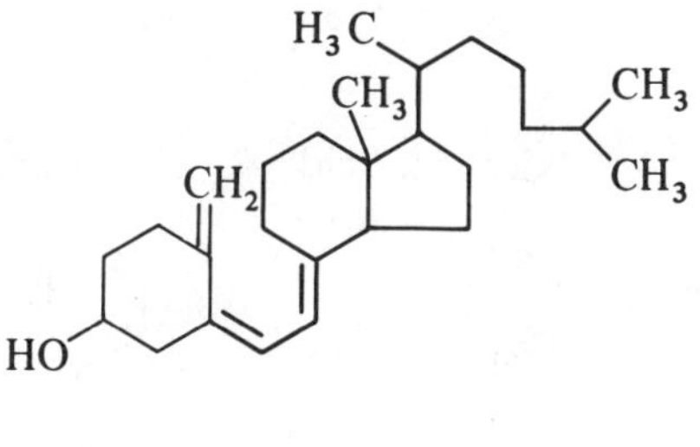

Vitamin A (retinol)

Nutritive Additives (*continued*)

Vitamin E (tocopherol) – R^1, R^2, and R^3
can be CH_3 or H in a number of combinations

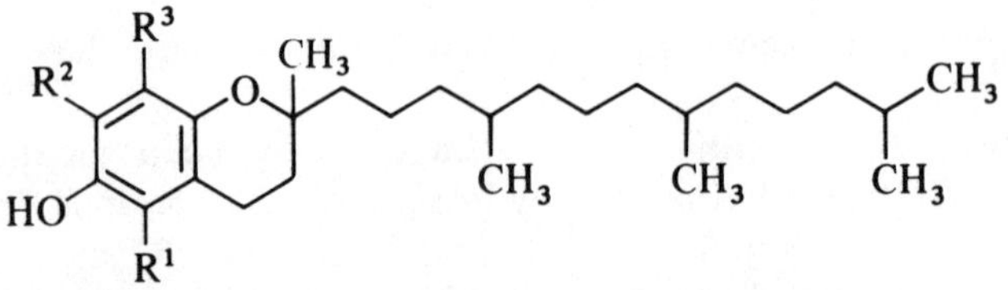

Vitamin K (bacterial origin)

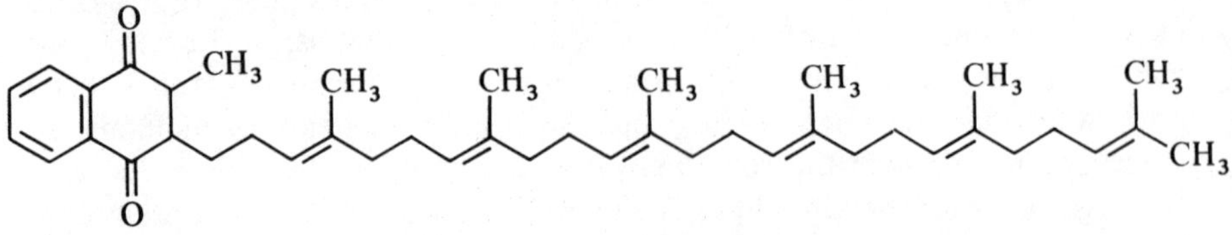

fat-soluble and require fat in the diet to be properly absorbed. The vitamins now to be described are all water soluble. For the most part they are precursors for (that is, they can be changed to) substances involved in the mobilization of biological energy by the metabolism of carbohydrates and fats. It follows that they act in concert with enzymes.

The principal water-soluble vitamins are thiamine (vitamin B_1), riboflavin (vitamin B_2), nicotinic acid/nicotinamide, pyridoxine (vitamin B_6), biotin and folic acid. It is worth noting that, like vitamin K, the normal source of

Riboflavin (vitamin B_2)

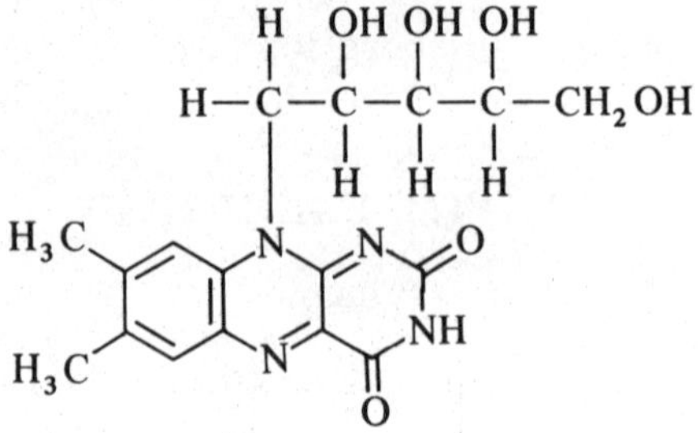

Nicotinic acid

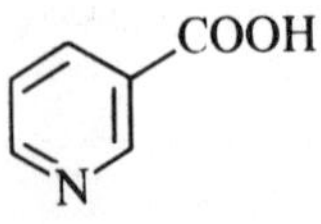

Nicotinamide

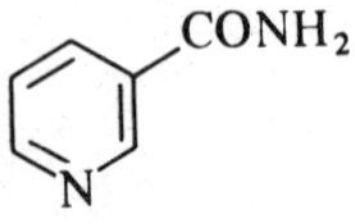

Pyridoxine

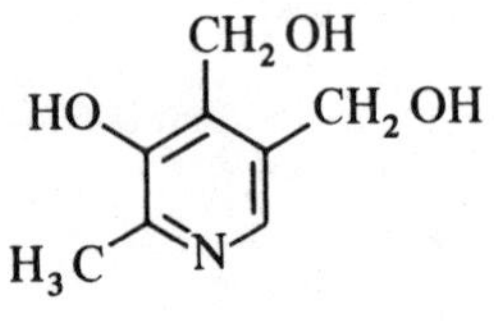

Nutritive Additives (*continued*)

Thiamine (vitamin B$_1$)

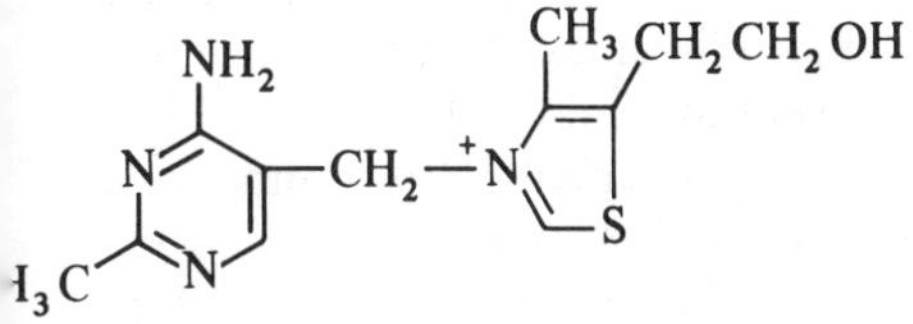

Pantothenic acid

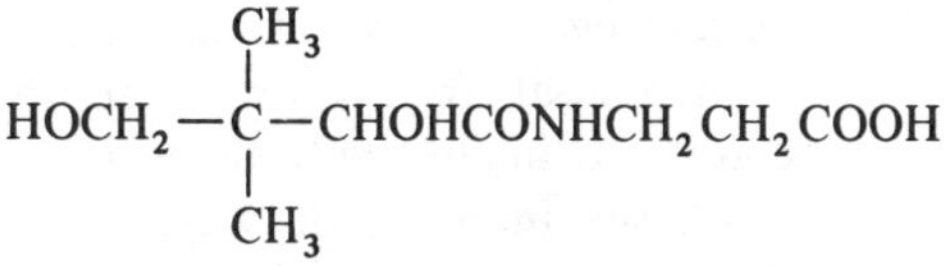

$$HOCH_2-\underset{\underset{CH_3}{|}}{\overset{\overset{CH_3}{|}}{C}}-CHOHCONHCH_2CH_2COOH$$

Biotin

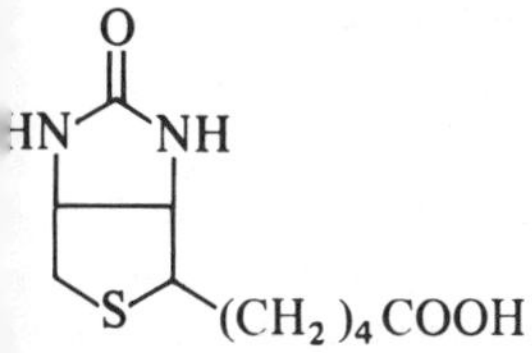

Folic acid

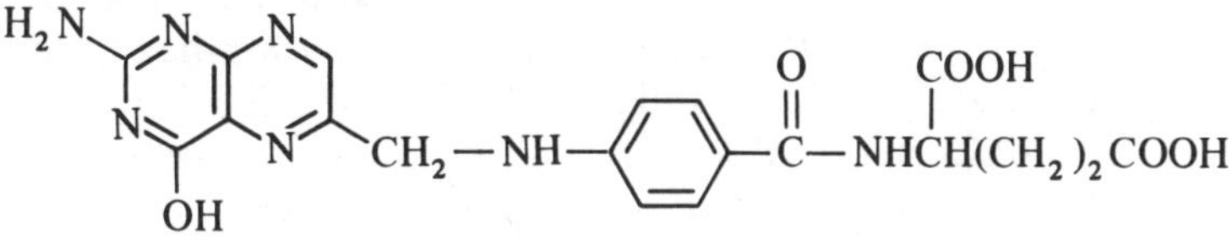

supply of a number of these vitamins is bacterial activity in the intestines.[47] Furthermore, insofar as antibiotics do not distinguish between alien and beneficial bacteria, anyone taking them should supplement their intake of the relevant vitamins to compensate for this.

Thiamine is a substance which, when in insufficient supply, gives rise to beri-beri: a disease common to countries where polished rice is a major article of diet. The vitamin is active only in the form of thiamine phosphate, in which form it is involved in the breaking of carbon–carbon bonds in carbohydrates. Absence of it leads to an excessive accumulation of pyruvic acid in the system and this is the immediate cause of the disease. It leads progressively to loss of appetite, nausea, neuritis due to degeneration of the nerve sheath, muscular convulsions, and cardiac disturbance. The body has no storage site for the vitamin and so there must be a regular supply. It is present in growing plant tips, in seeds and the outer coat of grains, and in wholemeal flour. It is added to white flour.

Riboflavin is one member of a large family of flavins which, characteristically, have a heterocyclic nitrogen-containing ring system coupled to a sugar group. The vitamin must be converted to a nucleotide before it becomes active. It then acts as a coenzyme, that is, in concert with an enzyme, for systems that are concerned with either, oxygen, hydrogen, or electron transport. The vitamin is produced in the plant world by germinating seeds and growing shoots, and in man by intestinal bacteria. Whether ingested or inbred, it is transported from the gut to the mitochondria—known as the power houses—of biological cells to take part in the production of energy. Deficiency symptoms are inflammation of the tongue, lesions at mucocutaneous junctions of the eyes and lips, congestion of conjunctival blood vessels, and desquamation of the skin.

Its constitution is such that its physical appearance is that of a bright yellow pigment, and for this reason it, and a phosphate derivative of it, are permitted food colours.

Pyridoxine is an unusual vitamin in the sense that, although there are deficiency symptoms in animals, and particularly in chickens, there are none in man, apart from general debility. It is present in seeds and grains and it is converted in the body to derivative forms that are involved in amino acid syntheses in a major way, both in decarboxylation (removal of carbon dioxide from intermediate compounds) and in transamination (transfer of amino groups from one acid to another). A number of the essential amino acids discussed later take part in transamination, and if they are in short supply the body will go out of nitrogen balance. So here we have a vitamin that we know is needed because we know what it does, and not because there are clearly identifiable ill effects if it is missing.

L-Ascorbic acid (vitamin C) is a simple unsaturated sugar lactone (see formula in the section on antioxidants) with remarkable properties for so simple a compound, and so unique for a sugar lactone. As a vitamin its basic role is to take part in a reversible oxidation–reduction reaction, and one of its specific jobs is to facilitate the conversion of the amino acid proline to hydroxyproline in newly forming collagen in tissue growth. For this reason it is always to be found mobilized at the seat of a wound. Gross lack of the vitamin leads to scurvy, common to seamen in earlier days. It is present in the growing tips of plants, the curative use of which the Chinese discovered many centuries ago. Fruits and vegetables are common sources today, but these are seasonal, and so the synthetic product is much used.

Pantothenic acid is another relatively simple compound, and it is normally well distributed in the diet, so that it rarely needs supplementing. It is essential for the formation of a key substance, coenzyme A, which takes part in the metabolism of both fats and carbohydrates. Here again there is no specific deficiency disease; only generalized symptoms of loss of appetite, restricted growth, and inflammatory lesions in the intestines.

On the other hand, cobalamin (vitamin B_{12}) is a very complex compound with a well-defined deficiency disease. It is so complex[42] that we will not attempt to give its formula here. Suffice to say that its function is to provide a source of cobalt. The deficiency disease is pernicious anaemia, which is one of arrested development of red blood cells. Normally the vitamin is supplied by bacterial synthesis in the intestines, though this implies an adequate supply of cobalt in the diet. However, there is sometimes a digestive malfunctioning that prevents the vitamin being mobilized and transferred to the liver. The malfunction is not capable of correction and the vitamin must be administered if the disease is to be controlled. Identification of its constitution, which made synthesis possible, was the first major triumph of X-ray analysis.

Ruminants develop a similar condition if the pasture is deficient in cobalt, but the precise role of the element has not yet been determined.

Biotin is yet another vitamin produced by intestinal bacteria. Normally there is no deficiency, but cobalamin is involved in its synthesis and obviously a shortage of one would lead to a shortage of the other. It acts as a cofactor in a number of enzymic carboxylase systems. A mild deficiency leads to dermatitis symptoms: extended deficiency to nervous disorders.

Folic acid is our final water-soluble vitamin, and it is again produced by intestinal bacteria. This is the normal supply for humans, though it is also present in green leaves, and was in fact first identified there. This is understandable for it plays a part in the biosynthesis of porphyrin, which is a particular organic structure designed to hold a metal atom: magnesium in the case of chlorophyll, cobalt in the case of vitamin B_{12}, and iron in the case of haem. It is not surprising, therefore, that a shortage of folic acid can lead to pernicious anaemia.

Trace Elements

Certain elements are necessary to a truly balanced diet, albeit at only trace levels. Whether they appear naturally in the diet is a matter of chance, depending on whether they were present in the soil in which the food was grown or the vegetation that animals grazed, and the extent to which plants or vegetation absorbed from the soil. It is a well-known botanical exercise to recognize specific elements in the soil by the wild plants that flourish there, and a matter of record that some plants will absorb specific elements preferentially to the point that they present a toxic risk to animals. Humans can minimize the risk that they may ingest too little or too much of the trace elements only by diversifying the sources of supply. In fact, the whole matter of requirements and supply is in a comparatively elementary state at present. However, there are some essential elements that are so widely distributed, and required at such low levels, that special techniques have had to be designed to show that they are in fact essential. They are chromium, tin, vanadium, fluorine, nickel, and silicon. As such, they do not come under consideration as possible additives.

Those that may be in short supply are iron, copper, manganese, molybdenum, selenium, cobalt, zinc, and iodine.

A shortage of iron leads to anaemia. It is needed for all haem groups and, in this and in other forms, it takes part in the transport of oxygen, in oxidation–reduction processes, and in the destruction of biological peroxides.

Copper also has a number of roles. It catalyses processes in which hydrogen is coupled to oxygen. It acts with iron to correct a particular anaemic condition. It takes part in the cross linking of collagen. A shortage leads to skeletal lesions.

Manganese is a cofactor for enzymes that facilitate the transfer of phosphate and hydroxy groups. It also takes part in dehydrogenation (removal of hydrogen) and peptidase (making or breaking of peptide links in proteins) processes. The most specific deficiency symptom is skeletal abnormality.

Molybdenum acts with flavin compounds, referred to earlier when dealing with riboflavin, in respiratory processes, i.e. processes leading to the formation of carbon dioxide and water through control of oxygen, hydrogen, and electron transport. However, if soil is over-rich in molybdenum, it can lead to copper deficiency in animals grazing the pasture.

Cobalt, as we have seen, is an essential component of vitamin B_{12}. The U.S. tends to discount the importance of the element *per se* because its only known biological use is in the form of the vitamin. But, if intestinal synthesis is to proceed, it is necessary that the reserves of cobalt should be adequate.

Zinc is a component of insulin, which controls diabetes; but it is also—like manganese—involved in specific dehydrogenation and peptidase processes. A shortage produces dermatitic effects. High phytate and fibre levels interfere with the absorption of zinc and this has led to a disturbed growth pattern in Middle East populations.

Iodine is needed for the biosynthesis of the hormone, thyroxine, from the amino acid, tyrosine. A minor deficiency leads to goitre: a major one to dwarfism and mental retardation.

Selenium deficiency cannot be considered apart from vitamin E and the link between them was discussed earlier. The seleno-enzyme referred to there is glutathione oxidase, and its function is to inhibit the haemolysis of red blood cells, that is, the swelling and bursting of the cells due to an osmotic inflow of water. It acts by maintaining the integrity of the membrane.

Minerals

Dietary substances classed as minerals are those elements required at greater than trace levels; though two of them, iron and magnesium, also have trace element roles. Iron, in fact, is a borderline case and it has been dealt with already as a trace element. The other dietary minerals are calcium, phosphorus, sodium, and potassium.

Magnesium, in its role as a trace element, acts as a cofactor with enzymes that hydrolyse polyphosphates. As a mineral it takes part in bone formation but just how it does this is not known.

Calcium—with phosphorus—provides the main substance of bones and teeth, hydroxyapatite, which is a hydrated calcium phosphate. It also plays a part in the nervous system, in the clotting of blood, and in heart and muscle action. It cannot be mobilized from the diet in the absence of vitamin D.

Phosphorus acts with calcium as described in the previous paragraph. It is also required for a variety of other metabolic processes. Some vitamins, for example, are active only as phosphate derivatives, while the adenosine phosphates are used to provide a storage system for biological energy produced by metabolism of fats and carbohydrates within the body.

Potassium and sodium provide important cations to regulate osmotic equilibrium between cells and the surrounding plasma. Potassium ions are concentrated within the cells and sodium ions without. There is a turnover in both that must be made good but, additionally, those taking diuretics to maintain a satisfactory water balance within the body are likely to find their sodium/potassium balance upset by loss of potassium, and this must be corrected.

Essential Amino Acids

When dealing with enzymes earlier, some description was given of amino acids and their incorporation in proteins. It was also stated that humans could not make from their own resources all the amino acids they needed to fabricate the multitude of proteins required for an active and healthy human organism. This missing ones must therefore be present in the dietary intake, and they are called essential amino acids. There are 8 of them out of a total of 20 that are used. The FAO/WHO have worked out desirable levels of each in terms of the overall protein intake, and have chosen to express this as mg of essential acid per g of protein, in terms of the nitrogen content, i.e. mg/g N. The levels are shown in Table 6.[44]

All but lysine and threonine are used in the transamination processes

Table 6. Desirable levels in body
of essential amino acids

Amino acid	mg/g N
Valine	270
Isoleucine	270
Leucine	300
Threonine	180
Lysine	270
Methionine	140
Phenylalanine	180
Tryptophan	90

ESSENTIAL AMINO ACIDS

Valine

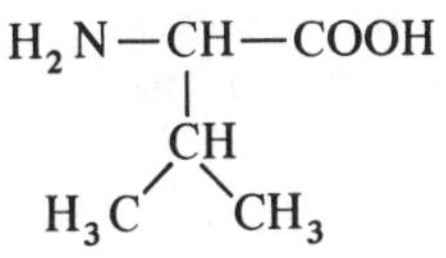

$$H_2N-CH-COOH$$
$$|$$
$$CH$$
$$H_3C \diagup \diagdown CH_3$$

Isoleucine

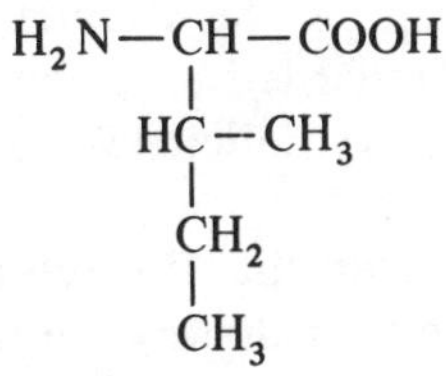

$$H_2N-CH-COOH$$
$$|$$
$$HC-CH_3$$
$$|$$
$$CH_2$$
$$|$$
$$CH_3$$

Leucine

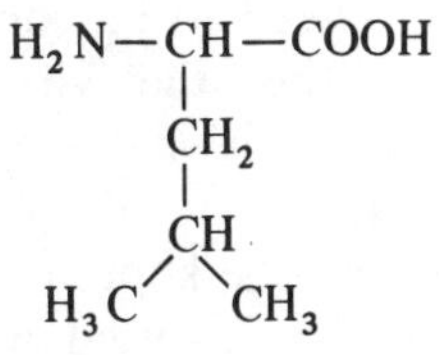

$$H_2N-CH-COOH$$
$$|$$
$$CH_2$$
$$|$$
$$CH$$
$$H_3C \diagup \diagdown CH_3$$

Essential Amino Acids (*continued*)

Threonine

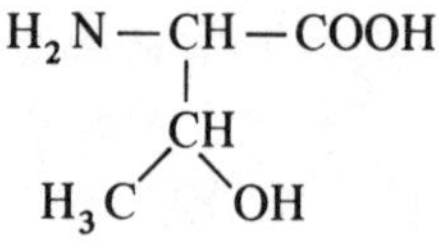

$$H_2N-CH-COOH$$

CH

H_3C OH

Lysine

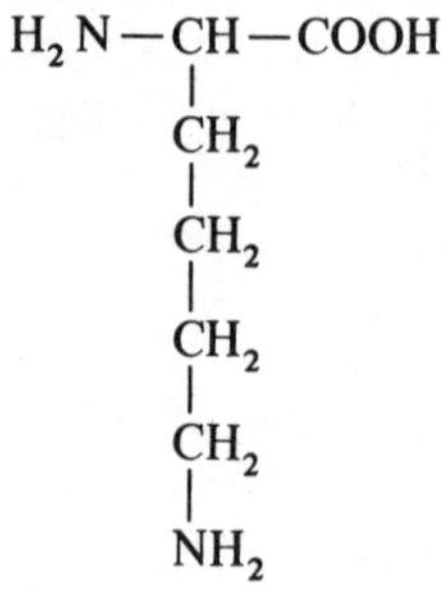

$$H_2N-CH-COOH$$
$$CH_2$$
$$CH_2$$
$$CH_2$$
$$CH_2$$
$$NH_2$$

Methionine

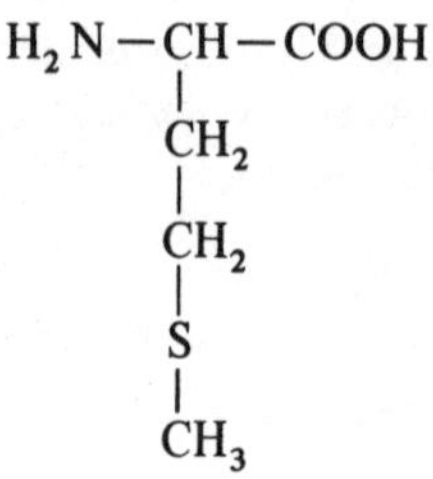

$$H_2N-CH-COOH$$
$$CH_2$$
$$CH_2$$
$$S$$
$$CH_3$$

Phenylalanine

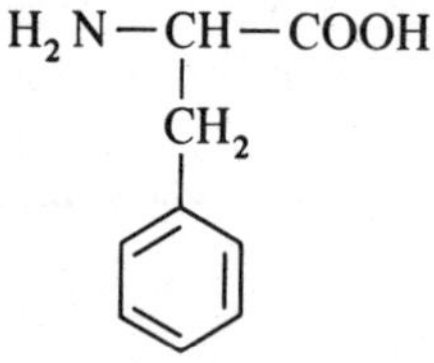

$$H_2N-CH-COOH$$
$$CH_2$$

Tryptophan

$$H_2N-CH-COOH$$
$$CH_2$$

N
H

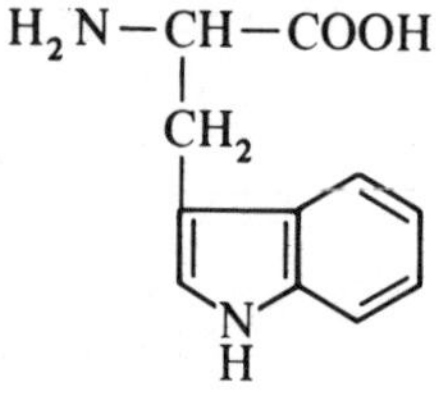

referred to when dealing with the vitamin, pyridoxine, earlier. Among the sources of protein in commonest use for food, the acids most likely to be in short supply are lysine, methionine, and tryptophan, with isoleucine on the borderline. Unfortunately tryptophan is the most difficult of the amino acids to estimate, and results must be viewed with caution. Lysine is low in wheat, corn, oats, rice, potatoes, groundnut, sunflower, sesame, and rape, methionine in wheat, oats, peas, soya bean, groundnut, cottonseed, and rape, and tryptophan (keeping the reservation in mind) in corn, beans, peas, and potatoes.

So far as U.K. control of vitamins as additives is concerned the following comment[45] is relevant.

'In general, the vitamins A, B_1 (thiamine), B_2 (riboflavin), nicotinic acid, C (ascorbic acid) and D are those of the most importance to the nutritionalist. However, folic acid and pyridoxine may possibly need to be considered among the vitamins of nutritional interest. The other vitamins are regarded as being of medical rather than nutritional interest as dietary deficiencies are so rare.'

It must be kept in mind, however, that this refers to the British scene where the diet is varied and the need for dietary control is fairly well understood.

In third-world countries much stricter control is required and greater understanding of what the available diet provides is needed before a similar situation is attained.

Fortunately the body is a very accommodating organism. There has to be gross underfeeding of any one micronutrient for evident symptoms to appear, and gross overfeeding to promote a toxic symptom (there is a case of a young man dying through an addiction to carrot juice) so that, although there are optimum levels for each micronutrient, some variation is possible without serious effect. Furthermore, what is optimum is a matter of periodic reassessment as fresh knowledge emerges. This is certainly true of vitamin C, and so far as vitamin K is concerned—and also for such trace elements as were discussed above but do not appear in Table 2 in Chapter 1—no recommended daily allowances (RDA) have yet been worked out. And even where there are RDAs for trace elements it would be difficult to organize diets to guarantee them because of the fortuitous nature of occurrence. So, for them, the table can be used, either as a guide for dietary use, or as a worksheet for supplementation.

So far as essential amino acids are concerned, it may be possible to provide a mixture of protein sources, as in the addition of soya flour to white flour, to ensure a reasonable supply but, since all essential acids can be synthesized, it is also possible, when supplies of protein of suitable quality are restricted, to make up deficiencies; though there are, as yet, no directives on this. Nevertheless, the acids are named as additives in an American publication,[21] and six of them appear in the Japanese permitted list,[27] the missing two being leucine and phenylalanine, but this is the only evidence of actual use. By and large, it is left to the judgement of manufacturers whether or not to supplement a food product with selected essential amino acids.

Indeed, in much that happens in the area of nutritive additives, a manufacturer can make his own judgement, within the provision of his own country's food law on safety. The addition of vitamins A and D to margarine is a classic case of a manufacturer anticipating legal enactment. This holds whether fortification is carried out to replace nutrients lost in processing, whether the product is in competition with others, or whether its purpose is to upgrade the product. In the U.K. there is legislation only when the product is in such wide demand as to make it a convenient vehicle for basic nutritional supplements, and we have already cited the examples of margarine and white flour. Infant foods are another example of intervention. Curiously, one has to consult, in the U.K., the Food and Drugs Labelling of Foods Regulations 1970[46] to find out which nutrients a manufacturer can claim credit for adding. What is even more curious is that there is no comprehensive report, either in the U.K. or the U.S., on nutritive additives; although, in the case of the U.K., there are such reports on other classes of additives. In the U.S. one can at least study the Federal Register and the Food Drug Cosmetic Law Reports to keep track of developments.

Flour and Bread Additives

All other sections in this chapter have been concerned with the various classes of additives used in large-scale food production or treatment. We end the chapter with comments of what is without doubt the most basic foodstuff of mankind, though it may be prepared in different ways and with different ingredients. Its basis is a cereal flour, and in western civilizations the product is principally wheaten bread. It may be a wholemeal bread, but there again it is more often a white bread made from treated flour.

The consequences of the large-scale demand for bread in terms of the additives required to maintain a wholesome product were dealt with in the closing paragraphs of Chapter 2, and these should be re-read at this stage. Here we are concerned with the characteristics of the substances required for the various additive roles. There are many kinds of bread of course, but by far the most popular is the white loaf, and comment will be limited to that.

In the U.K.[39] all flour must contain stated levels of chalk, iron (in a prescribed assimilable form), and the vitamins, thiamin and nicotinic acid (or nicotinamide). Both bleaching and improving agents are permitted in white flour, the former being defined as any substance capable of removing colour from ground bolted wheat, and the latter as any substance capable of simulating the effects produced by the natural aging of flour. Now the aging of flour is known to be the consequence of mild oxidation, so both classes of substances must be oxidizing agents, though their mechanisms must differ to undertake independent roles. Exergesists seem a little coy in differentiating between them, though one authority[40] does refer to the bleaching agent, benzoyl chloride, and the improving agents, L-cysteine hydrochloride monohydrate, ammonium persulphate $((NH_4)_2S_2O_8)$, potassium persulphate $(K_2S_2O_8)$, potassium bromate $(KBrO_3)$, chlorine dioxide (ClO_2), azodicarbonamide, and ascorbic acid. Ascorbic acid is the preferred improver for a specific breadmaking process which involves intense mechanical working of the dough.[41] We have met it already both as an antioxidant and as a nutritive additive.

FLOUR AND BREAD ADDITIVES

Benzoyl chloride

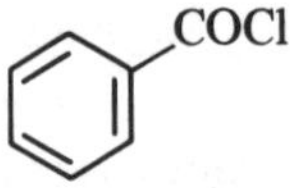

Azodicarbonamide

$$HN=C-N=N-C=NH$$

with OH below each C

Cysteine hydrochloride monohydrate

$$NH_2.HCl.H_2O$$

$$HS-CH_2-CH-COOH$$

Chlorine dioxide was admitted in place of nitrogen trichloride which was found to produce fits in dogs and so became suspect for man. It is likely that, in general, the choice of improver depends on the kind of plant used for breadmaking. It is to be noted that the FAO/WHO[19] also list acetone and nitrogen oxides.

Coming now to white bread, the U.K. regulations define it as composed of dough, made from flour, yeast, and water, which has been fermented and subsequently baked. It is permitted to contain any or all of: salt; edible oils and fats; milk and milk products; sugar; enzyme-active preparations; rice flour and soya flour. It is interesting that the U.K. authority which, as we have seen in the section on enzymes, is still considering the situation as a whole, should here have committed itself to permission to use enzyme-active preparations which it further identifies as malt extract, malt flour, amylases, proteinases, and lipoxidases.

Preservatives and emulsifiers/stabilizers have been considered generally in earlier sections. With respect to bread, the only permitted preservative, propionic acid, is unique to flour products. The choice is wider for emulsifiers/stabilizers, the following being permitted: mono- and diglycerides and certain esters of them; stearyl tartrate; sodium or calcium stearoyl-2-lactylate; naturally occurring lecithin. All these substances appear also in the FAO/WHO list.

CHAPTER 4

Legislative Processes

Legislative control of food additives is best seen as an extension of food control as a whole and, as such, so far as the U.K. is concerned, constitutes a continuing process whose origins lie far back in British history. But, because of the greater public awareness of happenings in the U.S.A., it is better to consider first the actions that have taken place there, and then to consider how other nations, including Britain, fit into, or contrast with, the U.S. legislative pattern.

American Practice

It has been said—and no one could contradict—that 'the American people have available the most abundant and variable food supply of any nation in history. This has been brought about in part by the application of science to food production and food technology'[30]. This is interesting, because the U.S. is largely, if not completely, self-sufficient in food supplies: unlike Britain, which is heavily dependent on food imports. It is well situated, not only to provide ample supplies of meat, grain, vegetables, and fruit for its own consumption, but also to have surpluses for export. Yet it is at the same time in the forefront in the development of processing and preservation techniques for conserving food, and also of promoting alternative sources of food, such as groundnut (peanut) and soya bean preparations.

In all this the Americans have remained clearly conscious of the implications of what they were doing, and the safeguards that must be maintained. Their approach may be summarized by a further quotation from the paper referred to above.[30]

'Many technological advances in food production have entailed the use of chemicals. Public awareness of the developments has focussed attention on the number and kinds of chemicals that enter food during production, processing, and storage. But statements that large numbers of chemicals are used in foods are uninformative and even misleading. It is necessary to know what the chemicals are, the extent to which they are used, and the foods to which they are added .... All components of food are chemicals classified as carbohydrates, fats, proteins, minerals and water. Foods also contain small amounts of accessory chemicals including the vitamins and antioxidants, antimycotics, buffers, thickeners, emulsifiers, chelating agents (sequestrants), colours and flavours.'

Although there was some sort of legal control in operation, as food technology grew in scope, a feeling grew that the situation should be reviewed, though stimulus for intensive official action did not develop till the 1950s. Prior to that, companies were supposed to know and avoid what was poisonous, and to restrict use of additives to substances of proven low toxicity; and thus ensure that they would be innocuous at the level required to obtain the desired product quality. Control in the modern sense started with the now historic Delaney Senate hearings during the 1950s. These culminated in 1958 in a Food Additives Amendment to the Federal Food, Drug, and Cosmetic Act of 1938. The Amendment set in motion two major policy changes with regard to additives. First, it replaced a 'policing' approach with one of 'licensing'. Second, it introduced the concept that for every chemical there is some finite level at or below which it can be present without prejudicing safety. Unfortunately, for reasons that are easy to understand but hard to justify, the concept was later modified to exclude substances that proved to be carcinogenic even though the level at which they had to be fed to produce the effect was grossly in excess of that at which they would be used.

We must now take note of what the Amendment meant when it used the word 'additive'. It is defined there as 'any substance that is, or may become, a part of food, if such substance is *not* generally recognised, among experts qualified by scientific training to evaluate its safety, as having been adequately shown to be safe under the conditions of intended use.' The contradiction with the yardstick for carcinogenicity will be immediately evident, but there is another contradiction that the Americans themselves recognize as peculiar.[15] It is that an additive defined above can never be allowed in food, whereas an additive which is *generally regarded as safe* (GRAS) under the conditions of intended use is no longer legally defined as an additive and can be used. However, anyone scanning the literature must not be misled by an occasional looseness of description. If that were the end of the matter permitted substances would be referred to simply as GRAS and discussion of American practice would be brief. Unfortunately, what happened before the Amendment was passed cannot be ignored and, after it, there were second thoughts that contributed their own measure of confusion.

Historically the first major piece of food legislation was the Pure Food and Drug Act of 1906, and this was followed in 1938 by the Federal Food,

Drug, and Cosmetic Act.[48] Both aimed generally to prevent the addition
of anything to food that might be poisonous or deleterious, but no specific
authority was named in the Act who could give approval for the use of
proposed additives. So, manufacturers wishing to make use of an additive,
did not proceed under the Act. Instead they applied to the Department of
Agriculture for a letter agreeing that food to which the substance was to be
added would not be rendered injurious thereby. This procedure was
continued by the Food and Drug Administration (FDA) for some time
following the passing of the Amendment, presumably till it could consider
the situation and organize its own procedures. These letters, which became
known as prior sanctions, became a source of some embarrassment when
improved methods of assessment were devised, and they are being
systematically withdrawn.

In brief, the system which the FDA inherited was one of permission
based on presumed safety which, in turn, was determined by absence of
either complaint or untoward consequences. On this the FDA had now to
superimpose, and in time replace with, a system requiring scientific proof
of safety. What it did at the outset was to consult with various scientific
groups 'comprising experts qualified by scientific training to evaluate
safety', and select a group of several hundred extant additives which, on
the available evidence, could be considered GRAS, and these were
published in the Federal Register, the Governmental official publication,
on 20 November 1959 and on 12 August 1960, in two parts. At the same
time it set in motion a new basis of judging proposed additives that were
not acceptable as GRAS. Such substances for which conditions of use
could be clearly identified, so allowing them to serve their intended
purpose at safe levels of addition, were to be regulated for use.

The Amendment did not name the FDA as arbiters in the matter. In
theory, it is left to any select group who can be recognized as 'qualified to
evaluate its safety . . . . under the conditions of intended use'. In practice
the FDA reserved the right to intervene, as we see from the following
quote concerning the use of vitamins and minerals.[49]

> 'A listing of some of the vitamins, minerals and compounds
> with vitamin and/or mineral properties which are generally
> regarded as safe (GRAS) and thus (since a substance which is
> GRAS is not a food additive, 21 U.S.G. 321(s)), lawful for use
> without a food additive regulation, appears at para 121. 101(d) (5)
> (21CFR121.101(d) (5)).
>
> As 21CFR121.101(a) specifically advises, it is impracticable to
> list by regulation all substances that are generally recognised as
> safe for their intended use. Accordingly, upon request, addressed
> to the US Food and Drug Administration . . . . it will advise
> whether, in its judgment, a particular use of a vitamin or mineral
> (not specifically governed by a regulation) is generally regarded as

safe within the meaning of 201(s) of the Act and thus lawful for use without a food additive regulation.'

So we see an element of judgment reserved by the FDA to determine whether something is GRAS or must be regulated. And indeed it had always been understood that any GRAS substance would be subject to review as any new evidence came to light. Nevertheless everyone was caught off balance when the cyclamate scare broke and its repercussions will be felt by the FDA for many years yet. But before we come to that we must return to the Amendment, or rather to the time of the hearings that led to it.

In view of the amount of work involved, and the direction in which the hearings were leading, the Food Protection Committee of the NAS/NRC assumed responsibility for compiling a list of additives in known use, and of the foods in which they were used: on a definition that was somewhat simpler than the one that emerged in the Amendment. It was that an additive substance, other than a basic foodstuff, that could be present in a food as a result of any aspect of production, processing, storage, or packaging. The Committee produced a short list of 517 substances during the hearings, in 1956, and a vastly extended list of around 4000 substances in 1965.[30]

We need not be astonished by the number however, for the greater part of the second list consisted of flavouring agents, and these included not only natural flavours, such as spices, herbs, tea, coffee, cocoa, strawberry, raspberry, lemon, orange, lime, and so on, but, also constituents of natural flavours. And, as anyone conversant with such composite substances will know, and as indeed we have indicated in the previous chapter, each may contain 50 or more constituents. Furthermore it is evident from a perusal of the list that investigators, having identified this or that substance as a constituent of a flavour, have synthesized many derivatives and analogues: variations on a flavour theme, as it were. Add to this that some substances, the long-chain fatty acids for example, seem to have slipped in under somewhat false pretences (they are edible but hardly flavoursome, as one understands the term) and it can be surmised that the basic list of flavours is rather less than half of those entered. Nevertheless it is not surprising to find, even now, a tendency to give low priority to scrutiny of flavour substances.

In fact, assessment of them, which—as noted in the previous chapter—could well daunt any review body, was passed initially to the U.S. Flavour and Extract Manufacturers Association (FEMA), which thereupon engaged a panel of six experts to assess the evidence. One thousand, four hundred substances came under review and, on the basis of identity, specification, test results, manner of use, and levels of addition, 1124 of these were judged to be GRAS. The FDA published the list in the Federal Register and thereby gave tacit consent to their use, but did not confirm them as GRAS. Indeed, it would seem that the FDA by now had decided in principle not to extend the GRAS list, but rather to proceed by regulation on a precisely defined basis as a means of official approval.

Such regulation would be issued only if:

1. The data supplied established that the proposed use was safe.
2. The proposed use would not promote deception of the consumer.
3. The additive would accomplish the intended technological effect.
4. The additive would not induce cancer when ingested by man or animal.

Matters appeared to be progressing smoothly on this basis when news broke in 1969 from a Canadian laboratory that the artificial sweetener, cyclamate, had produced cancer in rats, and cyclamate had already been approved as GRAS in the U.S. It had been used extensively in soft drinks and other products without adverse comment since the early 1950s. Use had been more restricted in the U.K., not from any suspicion of carcinogenicity, but because cyclohexylamine was liable to be produced as a by-product and no toxicity studies had been made on this. Indeed, in December 1967, control had been slackened to permit its use in any product other than ice-cream and bread. Now, with this adverse report, it was immediately banned in Canada and the U.S. and Britain quickly followed suit.

Action in the U.S. stemmed from a so-called Delaney clause in the Amendment which said that 'no additive will be deemed safe if it is found to induce cancer in man or animal, or if it is found, after tests which are appropriate for the evaluation of food additives, to induce cancer in man or animals.' It could be argued that, within the context of all that has been said, tests appropriate for the evaluation of food additives would lead to assessment at the levels of intended use. But insofar as the phrase has not been inserted in the Delaney clause, it has been held literally to be not applicable. So, while the Amendment in general is concerned with safety under conditions of use, cancer, as an emotive subject, is treated as a special case. The report that led to the ban showed that 10% of a colony of rats fed a mixture of cyclamate, saccharin, and glucose, in the proportions used in soft drinks, but at grossly exaggerated levels, had developed bladder cancer.

As interpreted by the FDA, the Delaney clause permitted no interpretation of findings, or use of judgment, no matter how extensive human experience might be on the matter. If a test, at any dose level and for any period of time, was positive, then a ban must follow—or rather, that was the instant decision. In fact, debate of the decision has continued. The conditions under which cancer was produced in no way corresponded with conditions of consumption. Nor was it explained why saccharin was not equally suspect. In fact, a repeat test with saccharin alone, carried out subsequently in Canada, has produced a similar result. But saccharin has been used for over 60 years without challenge and would be very difficult to replace. So only Canada has banned it, and not all countries have followed the line on cyclamate.[50] It is still listed by FAO/WHO.[19]

In the overall span of legislative action, the banning of cyclamate, though dramatic, was no more than an isolated incident, but the consequence for the FDA was momentous, for a Presidential decree followed that the FDA should initiate a complete safety review of all food additives then in use, including those in the GRAS lists. This meant that the schedule for examination of all previously approved substances had to be updated, not only to provide more specific assurance that any one additive would not cause cancer or chronic disease, but also to ensure the absence of reproductive and mutagenic hazards, for the public had been alerted by now to hitherto unsuspected side effects of certain drugs. The possibility that wholly original additives might carry similar risks could not be ignored.

The ensuing programme,[51] designed to replace the former *ad hoc* assessment, consisted of five parts:

1. A continuing review of the uses of non-flavour ingredients which had been classified as GRAS.

2. A safety review of direct food additives, other than flavours, which had been regulated by the FDA since 1958.

3. A safety review of all flavours, including spices.

4. A review of all provisionally listed colour additives.

5. A laboratory assurance programme.

It is worth noting the separation of flavours and colours from other additives, underlying the individual problems presented.

The programme has entailed four sequential phases:

1. A literature search covering 50 years to collect safety information, and an industrial user survey to establish customer exposure, for every substance. (Responsibility for the user survey was delegated to the NAS/NRC.)

2. All data to be collated and presented as a review.

3. Evaluation by expert food additive safety scientists to determine for each substance whether it can be generally regarded as safe, or whether it would require some limitation in the interests of safety.

4. A statement of proposals and final regulations to give official recognition of the re-evaluations.

It was implicit in the programme that the FDA hoped that for many substances sufficient new evidence would turn up for decisions to be made without further testing. It recognized, however, that such was the number of substances to be reviewed that there must be priorities. So, of the very many GRAS substances, 675 were selected for immediate attention, and of these 439 were non-flavours. It was decided either to have evaluations carried out by contract with the Federation of American Societies for Experimental Biology (FASEB), or to proceed by a mechanism of GRAS affirmation by petition, the FDA to decide which procedure to be adopted in each case.

The same kind of procedure was set up for the 400 or so non-flavour substances that had been approved by regulation since 1958. In a sense this had to be a running programme to accommodate substances also in the pipeline.

So far as the multitudinous flavour substances were concerned, a cloud of uncertainty developed on how best to deal with them. Two hundred and thirty-six of the selected GRAS substances were flavours and another 943 had been regulated by 1967. An inferential method of assessment was in use, but this needed now to be reviewed in the light of the Presidential decree. The whole matter has been delegated to the FASEB for study and recommendation.

A different kind of cloud hovers over colour additives, for reasons discussed in the previous chapter: an emotive cloud that has strongly influenced the criteria by which a colour might be permitted. So a provisional list of permitted substances has been drawn up, whose members might or might not appear in a permanent list when the stringent conditions for acceptance have been applied.

It is not for this book to attempt any kind of analysis of the consequences of this programme, but it is permissible to make some comment on it. First, there must be some common-sense judgment used in coming to decisions. The cost of comprehensive toxicological testing for a single compound has been put recently[52] at $500,000, and the time required at 3–10 years. It is evident therefore that, wherever possible, re-evaluation should be made on the basis of the 50 year literature search for existing data. Even on that basis it has taken 7 years, and cost 18×10^6 dollars to review just half of the non-flavour GRAS substances, and it has been calculated that it will take 4 years and cost 3.3×10^6 dollars for the more comprehensive testing required for just 8 of the provisional list of colours.It is unlikely that processors will submit claims for new additives unless there is clear evidence of marked improvement in the product and financial cover for the use of the additive.

To summarize as best we can, the use of food additives in the U.S. is controlled by a Food Additives Amendment of 1958 to the Food, Drug and Cosmetic Act of 1938. Control is exercised by the Food and Drug Administration (FDA). A broad permission to use, subject to good manufacturing practice, is granted if there is evidence to support the view that a substance can generally be regarded as safe (GRAS) under the proposed conditions of use. A narrower permission to use can be given in the form of a regulation which defines closely the conditions of use. By a quirk of definition, GRAS substances are not additives within the meaning of the Amendment: regulated substances are. In practice they all are. The situation contains ambiguities which, when they intrude, are resolved by FDA decision whether a substance is GRAS or must be subjected to regulation.

Current activities are in a state of flux due to the cyclamate scare of 1968 when the substance, hitherto listed as GRAS was reported to produce cancer in experimental rats. All listed substances, whether GRAS or regulated, are in a process of re-evaluation.

British Practice

Two points may be made at the outset vis-a-vis American practice. One is that, whereas in the U.S. it is sufficient that a substance is proved safe under the conditions of intended use, and that there is some evident advantage in so using it, in the U.K. there has also to be some particular need for it, that is, one not served by an already permitted additive. Hence in the U.S. there is a wider variety of choice and overall use is spread over a larger number of substances, while in the U.K. choice is more restricted and there is a greater use of fewer substances.

The second point is that additives in the U.K. like the British Constitution, are not defined in law. Instead, they are identified by purpose, such as flavouring, colouring, sweetening, and so on. What is defined is food, and this is stated in the definition to include 'articles and substances used as ingredients in the preparation of food'. In other words, independent consideration of additives is a matter of convenience only. In law they are all a part of food. Nevertheless, it introduces a certain ambiguity in that additives, by implication, are considered as ingredients, and in fact the two words are often used indiscriminately in official reports. Indeed there are those who would prefer to use the word ingredients to avoid the obloquy that has become attached to additives. However, to most people, ingredients and additives have quite different connotations, and we shall use the word additive consistently here.

The earliest known legislation concerning food was an Act of 1266[53] designed to prevent the selling of short-weight bread and of unsound meat. It was not very effective, nor were various other statutes issued hopefully—and intermittently—during the following seven centuries. Some were designed to help the mediaeval Guilds in their fight against such frauds of adulteration as adding dust to pepper, peaflour to mustard, roast corn to coffee, and hops to beer. It is interesting to see that what is now considered an improvement to beer was once branded as adulteration.

In spite of all these legislative activities, a situation was reached by the mid-nineteenth century that has been described as appalling. This led to the setting up of a select committee to consider the matter, and to the subsequent passing of an Adulteration of Food and Drinks Act 1860. Unfortunately, enforcement of the Act fell to local authorities and there was neither the finance available nor the will to act. A strengthened Adulteration of Food, Drinks and Drugs Act of 1872 aimed to help authority and supply expertise for the operation of it, particularly in the analytical field, but it was only partially effective.

Hope of really effective control came with the passing of a Sale of Food and Drugs Act of 1875, which stated unambiguously for the first time that 'no person shall sell to the prejudice of the purchaser any article of food or anything which is not of the nature, substance or quality demanded by such purchaser.' Heavy penalties were provided for, and yet, it was not until 1900 that it could be claimed that bread, flour, tea, and sugar were wholly freed from the machinations of dishonest traders. It is against this background of persistent dishonesty that one has to view any attempt to control additives.

With adulterants under reasonable control it was possible to give greater attention to those that masqueraded as additives, and in 1925 an order was made prohibiting the use of preservatives in food other than specified products, and stipulating that such additives should be identified on the label. The order was consolidated in 1928 in a new Food and Drugs (Adulteration) Act. The situation was reviewed yet again ten years later and a Food and Drugs Act (1938) passed into law. This was updated in 1955 for England and Wales and the updated Act is still in force, though currently (1978) under review. Parallel Acts were passed, for Scotland in 1956, and for Northern Ireland in 1958.

Under these Acts Ministers have power to make regulations that are legally enforceable 'in the interests of public health or otherwise for the protection of the public.' The Ministry of Agriculture, Fisheries and Food (MAFF) is responsible for preparing regulations concerning composition and labelling, and the Department of Health and Social Security (DHSS) for those concerning hygiene. Both work through committees, the MAFF having a Food Standards Committee (FSC) and a Food Additives and Contaminants Committee (FACC). The DHSS has a Committee on Medical Aspects of Chemicals in Food, and this in turn has a subcommittee that considers the toxicity of chemicals in food, consumer products, and the environment. The nutritional additives—vitamins, minerals, and trace elements—are the responsibility both of the MAFF and of the DHSS. Food labelling, however, which covers nutritional claims, is the responsibility of the FSC; while vitamins used in other roles, e.g. ascorbic acid as an antioxidant or riboflavin as a colouring agent, are dealt with by the FACC.

The FACC was set up in 1964 to lighten the load of the FSC which, till then, had included additives and contaminants within its responsibilities. Both Committees consist of independent experts drawn from both academic and industrial research backgrounds, but all serve as individuals and not to promote sectional points of view. Furthermore, to limit the chance of stagnation there is a regular turnover of committee membership, each serving for three years, and one fifth of the Committee retiring each year. The Chairmen are also independent and usually academics. The secretariat is supplied by the Ministry.

The FACC's brief is 'to advise the Minister of Agriculture, Fisheries and Food, The Secretary of State for Social Security, the Secretary of State for Scotland, and, as respects Northern Ireland, the Head of the Department of Health and Social Security, on matters referred to them by Ministers in relation to food contaminants, additives and similar substances which are, or may be, present in food or used in its preparation, with particular reference to the exercise of powers conferred on Ministers by Sections 4, 5 and 7 of the Food and Drugs Act 1955 and corresponding provisions in enactments relating to Scotland and Northern Ireland.'[54]

The FACC inherited from the FSC the dual tasks of reviewing substances already in use in the light of new evidence or requirements of evidence, and considering applications for new proposed additives. It is appropriate at this point to note two factors affecting their deliberations.

First, with respect to flavouring agents, the FSC had had these already under review and were to publish a report in 1965, that is, in the year following the setting up of the FACC. In that same year, moreover, the Council of Europe were to set up an *ad hoc* working party on Natural and Artificial Flavouring Substances[31] and to publish a report on its findings in 1974. This quite naturally influenced the FACC's own treatment of the matter.

Second, the UN FAO, in cooperation with the World Health Organisation (WHO), following a conference on Food Standards in 1962, had established a Codex Alimentarius Commission. This in turn had set up a Joint FAO/WHO Expert Committee on Food Additives to act as an advisory body to the Commission. The reader will sense, therefore, that there was already multiple activity in the field and, not unnaturally, the FACC took all this into account when making its own assessments.

As we have seen, interpretation of the wording of the 1955 Act has led the U.K. authority to proceed on the basis of grouping according to purpose, a system that has made it easier to ascertain whether a new submission was something different from, or identical in action to, something already permitted. The aim of the FACC is to produce statutory permitted lists for all groups of additives, and such lists now exist for antioxidants, emulsifiers, stabilizers, preservatives, colours, flavours, and a number of other groups dealt with in the previous chapter. At the same time the FSC have prepared companion product standards for additives in for example, bread and flour, butter, cheese, ice-cream, and soft drinks.

No list or product standard is considered immutable. All are submitted to review every five years or so and, if necessary, an amending regulation is issued. In carrying out a review, the Committee procedure is rather like that of the U.S. FDA except that, whereas the FDA commissions any necessary toxicological work from independent laboratories, the FACC does not. It carries out a critical examination of reports on work carried out since the previous review by Research Associations and by industrial and academic laboratories, and calls for evidence and submissions from all interested parties. Finally it issues a report of the review which carries recommendations of any changes deemed necessary.

So far as new submissions are concerned, there are guidelines on what is required and on the toxicological evidence to be offered in support of it.[55] In the U.K., testing is the responsibility of the company making the submission and, since this can be very expensive (in 1979 ranging from £250,000 to £350,000 for a fully comprehensive check), and the FACC has to be satisfied either that there is a technological need that cannot be satisfied by an already permitted additive, or that the need cannot be obviated by a change in production technique, it follows that need should be established as soon as possible, and certainly before the really expensive testing is undertaken.

In considering a submission, the Committee proceeds broadly as follows:

1. It considers the evidence supporting need: Why other existing additives are not suitable for the particular manufacturing process: In what way it serves the purpose better or is more economical: What advantage is offered to the consumer: Can its identity and purity be defined.

2. If need is accepted, the Committee considers the evidence of safety, and invites the views of the Coordinating Committee on Medical Aspects of Chemicals in Food and the Environment, and its specialist subcommittee on the Toxicity of Chemicals in Food, Consumer Products and the Environment. The evidence may well include:
    (a) Internal or sponsored research by the company making the submission.
    (b) Research carried out by the British Industrial Biological Research Association (BIBRA) or other research group. (BIBRA[56] is an organization financed by its member firms to undertake research of interest to all members.)
    (c) Recommendations of the Joint FAO/WHO Expert Committee on Food Additives.
    (d) Any other relevant information.

3. The Committee prepares a report setting out the evidence and findings, and includes in it a report of the Toxicity Sub-committee. The report may be expected to make one of four possible recommendations:

   (1) The submission should be rejected.
   (2) Further evidence of need or safety is required before approval can be given.
   (3) Temporary permission should be granted for a specific period, when a further review will be made.
   (4) Permission should be granted for the substance as specified, with prescribed limits of addition, and listed foods to which it is applicable.

Such a report does not commit the Ministers concerned, nor is it necessarily final, for it is open to representations and consultations by interested parties before final submission. If the report survives this scrutiny, either in its original form or after agreed modification, and the Ministers approve it, then it is passed to experts for the drafting of a regulation in that legalistic language so necessary to minimize misinterpretation, and so certain to hamper interpretation. If the regulation includes provision for labelling, description, or advertising, the Food Hygiene Advisory Council is consulted at this stage. The draft regulation, like the earlier report, is made available for representation and consultation before it is finalized as a Statutory Instrument under the Act and submitted to the Ministers for signature. It will be seen that no proposed additive is lightly or carelessly permitted for use.

European Economic Community Practice

Although there is a similarity in approach to the matter of additives among members of the Community, national idiosyncracies in food preferences, in appearance, quality, and flavour, and even in definition, pose problems. West Germany, for example, did not recognize 'food additives' as such, but only as 'foreign substances', and then adopted a definition that excluded substances of natural origin or substances that are chemically identical with natural substances, and are generally considered by the public as being used primarily because of their nutritional, olfactory, or taste values.[57] Such things do not ease the way of the EEC, one of whose aims is to harmonize practice among the nine member countries. The late admission of Denmark, Eire, and U.K. with their own well established practices, found them at variance with the original six, and Community directives have to take account of this. All this gives one an inkling of the difficulties in achieving greater uniformity in world practice.

The Community works through a Scientific Committee for Food whose members are either expert technologists, toxicologists, nutritionists. All are drawn from national specialist committees, such as the U.K. FACC, in order to maintain effective contact with policies and action in the individual countries. The method of working is to determine to what extent conformity of control is possible in any given additive in use in one or other country, or in some or all countries; to draw up a directive that the majority of countries can accept, and to indicate where necessary permitted divergences by particular countries. In such cases the directive will specify the period for which permission to diverge will apply, after which the situation is reviewed in the hope of reaching greater conformity. In this manner partial conformity has been reached on emulsifiers, stabilizers, thickeners, gelling agents, colouring agents, preservatives, and antioxidants.

A Community directive is not mandatory. It must be incorporated in a regulation for each country under its own Food Law. The U.K., as we have seen, operates under a law of 1955. Italy brought its law up-to-date in 1962, Denmark in 1973, and Belgium and West Germany in 1974. The French operate under a law of 1905 which was so worded as to permit subsequently a series of amending decrees that enable it to function as a modern food law. A description of the consultative procedures set up by the Community Commission is to be found in ref. 70, and a detailed summary of achievements in the field of food additives ref. 71.

Practice in Eastern Countries

We have information on practice in both India and Japan which, though incomplete, enables us to make some comparison with western practice. First, both countries work with much shorter lists of permitted additives, and second, both countries incorporate the additives, with conditions of use, in their Food Act. In the case of India this is the Prevention of Food Adulteration Act 1954 and in the case of Japan the Food Sanitation Law: Both laws, however, can be amended by way of regulation to admit new additives. The Japanese Act lists some ninety or so permitted flavours. The Indian Act merely records that coumarin and dihydrocoumarin are prohibited, and this presumably gives Indian manufacturers a very free hand. All further comment will be relative to the Japanese practice.

Japan, like Western Germany, classes additives as occurring naturally or of synthetic origin. But if one that occurs naturally is modified before use, or a synthesized form is used, it is classed as synthetic. Those classed as of natural origin do not need approval and listing before use, but those classed as synthetic do.[27] Investigation of proposed new additives is carried out by a Food Sanitation Investigation Council in accordance with relevant articles of the Food Sanitation Law.[58]

To obtain approval the applicant must show:

1. The additive is demonstrably safe.

2. The additive is advantageous to the consumer in that it satisfies one or more of the following conditions:
   (a) It is necessary to the manufacturing process.
   (b) It helps to maintain the nutritional value of the food.
   (c) It prevents or minimizes degradation of the food.
   (d) It increases the attractiveness of the food.
   (e) It reduces the price to the consumer.

3. The additive can be shown to be either superior to, or more useful than, existing registered additives.

4. The additive can be chemically identified by analysis in the food as sold to the consumer.

Factors that could lead to rejection are:

1. The additive could disguise poor quality in either the basic food or manufacturing process.

2. The additive could impair nutritional quality.

3. The purpose is either curative or therapeutic.

4. The desired improvement could be obtained by modifying the manufacturing process.

It may be noted that Japan deals with nutritional aspect of additives more explicitly than other countries, and indeed it seems to be only one that lists permitted nutritional additives.[27]

If the substance is not rejected at this stage, the applicant must then produce evidence of identity and specification, and of toxicological safety at proposed levels of use. For the latter, the testing must be done, either at two authentic research institutes in Japan, or at one such institute if reliable supporting evidence is available from foreign literature sources; the Council reserving the right to call for additional evidence if the situation so requires.

CHAPTER 5

Food and Agriculture Organization/World Health Organization Activities

We have seen in the previous two chapters how the developed world has dealt with the situation arising from an increasing need for food additives. We have now to give greater emphasis to the developing world and to the key role being played there by FAO/WHO.

It is to be noted at the outset that the position in developing countries is a confused one in which many bad habits of adulteration persist, and the authorities are as concerned to eliminate contaminants as they are to control additives. In this, former colonies, by and large, have the benefit of laws introduced by the colonial powers before secession. A number of African countries for example have laws similar to the U.K. Food and Drugs Act 1875, and some have updated the legislation. But the standard of control is very uneven, a major problem being the lack of skilled people to deal with it.

Furthermore, there are countries that lack any sort of control system, and there is a need here, given time and opportunity, to legislate for a basic food law that will take account of a country's resources of food and potential for food production. In the absence of legislation, some of these countries have required certificates from companies importing food to say that it complies with the law and standards of the country from which it came.

Finally there are countries whose legislation is so inadequate as to be almost worthless. Here the situation can be remedied only by a major overhaul, or by repeal and replacement of the existing legislation. This is where the FAO/WHO has a part to play.

The Food and Agriculture Organization of the United Nations and the World Health Organization are two bodies whose interests have overlapped to such an extent that they work jointly in many fields, and they are then known conjointly and succinctly as FAO/WHO. The WHO is the elder by some 18 years.

Many of the developing countries are food exporters, while the developed countries are importers with a standard of import control. It is in the common interest of both to maintain effective control. Recognizing this, the FAO/WHO commissioned a study of the guidelines that would be most useful in helping to set up an effective food control system for developing countries.[59]

The Guidelines, as finalized, were a blueprint to the setting up of a food control service: creating the service structure; devising a food law; developing food standards regulations; building up an administrative and laboratory service, and other ancillary aspects. The gist of the Guidelines' message was that, while offering the basis of food control, it was necessary for a food law to be enacted if the provisions of the system were to be enforced.

The Guidelines had this to say about the use of additives:

> 'The rapidly accelerating use of chemical additives such as antioxidants, preservatives, emulsifiers, colours and flavours, creates complex problems. Such use is stimulated by the need to:
>
> 1. maintain the physical and nutritional quality of food during shipment, storage and distribution;
> 2. make foods more attractive, more nutritious, or otherwise more desirable.

Some of these chemicals have been used in foods only recently. There is concern about the safety of many of these additives, particularly about chronic toxicity, mutagenicity, teratogenicity or carcinogenicity. Most countries exercise some control over the use of food additives.'

> 'From the point of view of national planning there should be recognition of the value food additives may have for preserving the physical and nutritional qualities of food, and for making them more attractive. Because of the dangers of uncontrolled use, however, legal controls are necessary. Failure to adequately control the use of additives in food can lead to rejection of shipments with consequent losses. Recommendations of the Joint FAO/WHO Committee on Food Additives can be helpful in this connection. To take advantage of this, appropriate legislation is needed.'

The preamble to the report on the Guidelines stated that it was part of a programme of support to accelerate or expand the work of the FAO/WHO Codex Alimentarius Commission on international standards for pollutants in food, and strengthen FAO/WHO capabilities to assist developing countries in food control. Thus it underlined the necessity of tackling adulteration as a primary step in any programme of food control. The examples given in the report of prevalent methods of adulteration were reminiscent of those occurring in Britain in the Middle Ages—sand mixed into salt; ash into spices; colour, flavour, and preservatives added to stale or decayed meat to make it appear fresh and of good quality.

The Codex Alimentarius Commission referred to above had been set up in 1962 to implement a Food Standards Programme.[60] The aim of the programme was to protect the health of consumers and ensure fair practices in the food trade world-wide by participating in and helping to coordinate food standards work among all bodies concerned with such matters. In practice this meant determining priorities and preparing standards with the help of other expert bodies, and publishing such standards as had attained overall approval among participating countries in a Codex Alimentarius. These standards would be applicable on either a regional or a world-wide basis. It was implicit in this that such standards were not necessarily absolute, but could be influenced by regional requirements.

Membership of the Commission is voluntary and over 100 countries now participate. The Commission has formed a subsidiary body to deal with additives, known as the Joint FAO/WHO Codex Committee on Food Additives, and this in turn has appointed a Joint FAO/WHO Expert Committee on Food Additives (JECFA). The parent Codex Committee is an inter-governmental body that meets periodically (one to one and a half years) to consider recommendation of the Expert Committee concerning levels of use of approved additives in specified foods, specifications for identity and purity, and methods of analysis for determination in food. It also prepares lists of additives for itoxicological examination by the Expert Committee. It reports to the Commission.

The JECFA consists of scientists who serve in a personal capacity. It evaluates additives referred to it on the basis of available data. It works out chemical specifications, establishes 'Acceptable Daily Intakes', (ADI), and examines toxicological data. The ADI, a term introduced by the Commission, is the amount for man that can be taken daily in the diet for a lifetime without risk. Unless otherwise stated all ADIs are expressed as mg/kg body weight. (Flour treatment agents are expressed as parts per million.) It is fixed at one hundredth of the maximum amount that can be fed to animals without toxic effects.

The Codex Committee considers these reports together with data supplied by member Governments, and prepares its own reports, with recommendations, for submission to the Codex Commission. In doing so. it checks:

1. that the toxicological tests take account of any cumulative, synergistic, or potentiating effects;

2. that the evidence presented makes it satisfactorily certain that the additive presents no health hazard at the proposed level of use;

3. that the specifications for identity and purity are acceptable;

4. that the additive will serve one or more of the following four purposes:

    a. it preserves the nutritional value of the food, unless the value is not significant in terms of the whole diet, or purpose 'b' that follows is more significant;

    b. it provides a necessary ingredient or constituent for foods manufactured for groups having special dietary needs;

    c. it enhances the keeping quality or stability of a food, or improves its organoleptic (i.e. flavour and taste) properties, provided that, in so doing, it does not deceive the consumer concerning the nature, substance, and quality of the food;

    d. it provides an aid to manufacture, processing, preparation, treatment, packing, transport, or storage of food, provided that, in so doing, it does not hide effects due to the use of faulty raw materials, or of undesirable practices or techniques.

The ADI may be qualified at this stage in the light of the Committee's study of the recommendations. Thus it may be given as 'not limited', 'not specified', 'conditional', 'unconditional', or 'temporary'.

    'Not limited' means that there is no explicit indication of an upper limit. It was assigned to substances of very low toxicity. It has now been superseded by 'not specified'.

    'Not specified' means that on the basis of available data the total daily intake required to achieve the desired effect does not represent a hazard to health. For this reason the establishment of an ADI is not deemed necessary. Its use, however, must conform to good manufacturing practice (GMP).

    'Conditional' is allocated when the Committee considers that the available data are inadequate for an unconditional ADI and further work is required, or if there are reasons arising from dietary requirements. The reasons for this and the restrictions imposed are stated in the evaluation.

    'Unconditional' is allocated to substances for which the biological data include favourable results of adequate long- and short-term toxicological studies and/or biochemical and metabolic studies. An unqualified ADI is classed as unconditional.

    'Temporary' means that there is insufficient data to establish whether or not a substance is toxic, and further evidence must be submitted within a stated period of time. Details are included in the evaluation. If the evidence is not produced in the stated time the ADI is withdrawn.

The Commission, which is responsible for the ultimate act of approval or disapproval, works to its own definition of additives. This is:

'For the purposes of the Codex Alimentarius, food additive means any substance not normally consumed as a food by itself and not normally used as a typical ingredient of the food, whether or not it has nutritive value, the intentional addition of which to food for a technological (including organoleptic) purpose in the manufacture, processing, preparation, treatment, packing, packaging, transport or holding of such food results, or may be reasonably expected to result (directly or indirectly) in it or its byproducts becoming a component of or otherwise affecting the characteristics of such food. The term does not include contaminants, or substances added to food for maintaining or improving nutritional qualities.'

When the Commission gives approval, either firm or temporary, for the inclusion of a substance in an advisory list, the approval is limited as far as possible to specific foods for specific purposes, and to the lowest level of effective use. It is based if possible on the ADI, or equivalent assessment, established for the additive, and the probable daily intake from dietary items of all kinds. It makes separate conditions of use for groups having special dietary needs. Any such approval rests on an understanding that the additive will be kept under surveillance and re-evaluated as necessary in the light of changing conditions of use or fresh scientific evidence.

Comparison of the criteria set out earlier with those of developed countries in the previous chapter reveals such a wide measure of agreement that one may wonder why there is such duplication of effort in determining the admissibility of any one additive, particularly as every authority is working towards the creation of positive lists, that is, lists which state which additives are permitted, and the conditions under which they are permitted. That there is duplication is a sign that judgement comes into the matter of approval and the factors which affect judgement vary from country to country. The considerable degree of conformity that exists, therefore, may be taken as a pleasing sign.

The importance of the Commission's work relative to that of other authorities is that it is intended primarily to help developing countries achieve control as effective as that of developed countries and, in so doing, facilitate international trade in foodstuffs to the benefit of the developing countries. The general pattern of procedure is the same whether the additive is intended for use on a regional or on a world-wide basis. It is set out in a procedural manual.[61] It involves preparing, in succession, a proposed draft standard, a draft standard, and a recommended standard; the second the third being the consequences of discussion on their predecessors. The work of drafting and redrafting falls on a subsidiary committee of the Commission set up for this particular purpose.

A proposal for a regional standard originates within member states of the region and, although discussion of the various drafts is wide-ranging among all member states, and even among outside specialist organizations, decisions are restricted to member states within the region, each of which can make reservations concerning application of the standard to its own country. (The reader will sense a similarity here to the working of the EEC.) Discussion of a proposed draft takes place by correspondence. Discussion on both draft and the recommended standard take place at appropriate sessions of the Commission and decisions are made there.

A proposal for a world-wide standard originates only within the Commission, and discussion on all drafts takes place by correspondence, the Commission deciding when there is sufficient concensus to make progress. Again, any state may make reservations concerning its adoption of the recommended standard.

The Commission publishes both categories of standards in the Codex Alimentarius when it considers that the weight of support justifies this. In doing so, it will list all those countries that accept the standard in total, and also detail all specified reservations, and the countries making them. This is very much regulation by consent, for as pointed out earlier, the Commission's work is wholly advisory, and requires a legal enactment in any country that wishes to make use of its work. Nevertheless the standing of the organization is such that no developing country dare ignore it when taking action on food control. And all developed countries take note of its findings when framing their own regulations.

CHAPTER 6

Safety Testing

The basic key to safety is the quality of testing. Given that, it will be seen from the previous chapter that the chance of any substance slipping through the inquisitorial net is minimal, and the periodic review implicit in all acceptances will provide an even tighter check. Twenty years ago it was different. Then the onus was on manufacturers to operate within the law as it was then framed and avoid evident toxic substances. Safety was assumed if the substance was found to have low toxicity and was incorporated at low levels in the food item. Control in the modern sense came with an escalation in the use of additives and was a consequence of the Delaney hearings in the U.S. which made evident a growing public desire for more definitive procedures for evaluating the safety of substances added to food products.

This in turn brought to the fore the need to define more exactly what is meant by safe, Paracelsus's famous remark—that all substances are poisons—has been noted and commented on in Chapter 1. Today, although all toxicologists are agreed that for even the safest food there is an upper limit of intake above which it will no longer be safe, they add that for all toxic substances there is a lower level in intake below which it will not have a toxic effect. Safety tests are therefore designed to show what these upper and lower limits are. In considering the tests, we will be more concerned with the aims that lie behind them, and the means whereby scientists set out to achieve those aims, than with the minutia of the tests themselves. For these the reference sources must be consulted. At the end of it all, however, it is the experience acquired of the consequences of human consumption of substances that have been permitted for use that will justify that permission.

It is to be observed at the outset that additives as such do not present a unique risk with respect to food intake, but that public concern has demanded that they be treated uniquely. Furthermore, it is also to be observed that in most matters related to living organisms one is not concerned with certainties but with probabilities. And indeed such a situation is not confined to the biological scene, for it holds also for social and political affairs. In scientific terms nothing is certain: all that can be said is that in some circumstances the degree of uncertainty is so low as to be discounted. It is when the evidence is elusive and difficult to interpret that probabilities are introduced to help define the situation in terms that will help in making a judgment.

One thing that might have been expected to help clarify the situation has, in fact, added to the confusion. It is that diagnostic techniques are becoming increasingly sensitive and are disclosing new potential risks where none were suspected before. And it has, in a curious way, drawn natural foods under greater scrutiny than hitherto. According to one reference,[62] of six classes of hazard associated with food listed there, that of natural toxicants ranks higher than that of additives, which are themselves held to present the least risk. It has to be recognized, however, that this is due in part to adopting 1% of a no-effect level as a permitted safe level, for this puts quite a number of common food constituents into the risk class. It is known, for example, that the limits between risk and benefit for such diverse but necessary substances as salt and vitamin A are much closer than this, and it is very likely that the play-safe level of 1% has been far too uncritically arrived at. This anomaly has to be removed and laboratories in general are moving towards it in terms of a decision-making tree to be discussed later.

We must return now for a moment to the subject of probability, to make the point that lay readers of this chapter should not be misled into thinking that the intrusion of probability diminishes the power of making a judgement. On the contrary, it increases it, for the manipulation of probability is a very exact mathematical science. What is important is that any experiment should be properly designed, so that all the data from it are significant. There can be a basic pattern for the experiment, but it must have the flexibility to satisfy particular requirements. Given all this, the experiment will provide a very good measure of the chosen parameter and of the limits of uncertainty to be attached to it. Our knowledge of vitamin requirements is rooted in biometric evaluations of this kind and, in turn, the biological basis of additive testing may be said to be rooted in vitamin testing.

It is in no small measure due to this that small animal laboratories have been in operation for the greater part of this century. In consequence, an expertise has been developed, and a fund of knowledge built up, on the applicability and use of small animals in work of this kind. Overall, rats and mice have been found to be the most useful experimental animals, not least because they require minimal laboratory space and have a relatively short life span, so that all eventualities can be covered in a reasonable length of time. Most animals that are used today are the result of special breeding over many generations, though this is not to say that wild types are ruled out. They have a use in the overall programme of testing.

Nevertheless the great majority are either inbred (that is, offspring of brother–sister matings over many generations), outbred, or crosses of inbred varieties. Inbreeding increases genetic uniformity and so minimizes variability of response to a test substance. Outbred animals or a cross of inbred, would be used if inbreeding had unduly decreased the sensitivity of the animal to the parameter being used to assess risk. If outbred, larger groups of animals would be required to allow for the greater variation in individual response. Crosses are a compromise. In all cases the basal diet, that is, the diet fed to controls, and to which the test substance is to be added for the experiment, must be so chosen that it does not obscure the effect that is being investigated.

Finally, since no one species of animal corresponds in biological response unambiguously to that of man, and humans cannot be used until risk is proved reasonably non-existent, a second, non-rodent, species may be employed in confirmatory toxicity tests. Overall, the following species of animals may be found within the stock-in-trade of any one laboratory: rodents—mice, rats, hamsters and guinea pigs: non-rodents—rabbits, chickens, ferrets, pigs, dogs, and primates.

Another important factor in obtaining significant results is the manner in which the animals are managed: a matter of miniature animal husbandry as it were, involving overall cleanliness of the laboratory, size and population of cages, manner of feeding and collection of urine and faeces, and so on. It is practised more rigorously in an animal laboratory than in any large-scale husbandry on a farm.

For mutagenicity testing, and particularly in screening tests, that is, tests designed to assess the likelihood of genetic toxicity, selected micro-organisms are used, which provide a rapid, cheap test and also because the chance of mutation is higher. Care has to be taken, however, not to include species with a high chance of spontaneous mutation.

Before any tests are carried out it is important to identify both the origins of the substance and its physical and chemical characteristics: this to ensure that, if it is cleared for use, what is subsequently used is identical with the test material. There must also be an assessment of the likely consumption by the public, and the extent to which children would be involved, to be taken into account when making a final recommendation.

The tests themselves cover two broad areas of possible ill-effects, insofar as they are concerned with acute, subchronic, and chronic toxicity on the one hand, and with carcino-, muta-, and teratogenicity on the other. Various ideas for a decision-making tree based on these have been made, but we will confine ourselves to just one of the suggestions since thay are all similar[62] (see p. 97).

It will be seen that although there may be grounds for rejection at any stage of examination, acceptance is possible only in the final stages. What is not so evident is the range of disciplines involved in reaching a decision. So these are listed below:

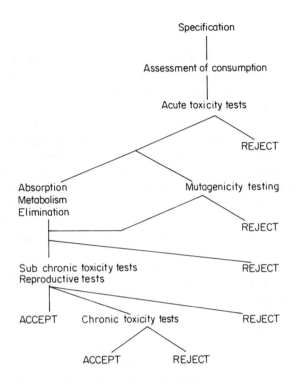

Chemistry: analysis of test substance.

Bacteriology: (or microbiology): screening for mutagenic acitivity.

Veterinary pathology: clinical examination, necropsy, histological examination.

Haematology: analysis of blood.

Biochemistry: metabolism in animals, analysis of excreta and body fluids.

Pharmacology: study of effect on organ function.

Immunology: study of ability to cause allergy.

Statistics: Analysis of data.

We are now ready to consider what the tests involve.

Acute Toxicity

The central purpose of this test is to assess the likelihood that the substance will cause death, and to determine the conditions under which it will do so, keeping in mind the maxim that all substances are potential poisons and it is the dose that determines whether or not it will be lethal. A subsidiary purpose is to provide a dosing guide for further tests if the substance survives the acute toxicity hurdle. Primarily, however, the test is designed to determine the amount of a substance which, when given as a single dose, may cause death; and since a large single dose is not necessarily a pointer to the effect of smaller doses repeated over a period, this test has little relevance to what is generally understood as safety evaluation.

In a typical test two rodent and one non-rodent species might be used, but a preliminary run may be made with a single species to get some idea of what the toxic dose for the substance is. Then, in the actual test, a range of doses is administered to groups of animals—orally by stomach tube—such that at one end of the range there are no deaths, and at the other there is 100% mortality, with three intermediate levels yielding between 16% and 84% mortality. If the substance has a very low toxicity, it will be necessary to administer repeated doses, albeit over as condensed a period as possible to approximate to a single dose, in order to induce a toxic response.

For ease of subsequent statistical treatment the dosages are spaced logarithmically but, for satisfactory dietary response, they are then diluted with a neutral carrier to equal volumes. There may be up to 10 animals of each sex in a dosage group, and they are observed for 2 weeks after dosage. The results are treated statistically to derive dose/mortality curves, and the dose likely to kill 50% of the animals is read off. This, the LD_{50} value, is the parameter for acute toxicity.

Genetic Toxicology

In order to understand genetic toxicology we must first put it into context by sketching in the macromolecular background to genetic processes. We start by reference to what is popularly known as the thread of life, the double-stranded deoxyribonucleic acid (DNA), each strand built up of alternate sugar (deoxyribose) and phosphate groups, and each sugar carrying one of four nucleotide bases as a side group (see p. 99). The bases are distributed along each strand in such predetermined manner that, first, each successive set of three bases is a code for an amino acid to be picked up and incorporated in a protein (most of these will be enzymes: see relevant section in Chapter 3). Second, the comparative sequence of bases along the two strands pair off in a set fashion as shown in the sketch to create the double strand. In the cellular process of division that is the basis of both growth and reproduction, the paired strands separate and duplicate to produce two identical paired strands.

The operative length of DNA is known as a chromosome and it is 'marked off' in the subunits known as genes, each of which is responsible for just one heritable factor in the living organism. Species characteristics are determined by the number and lengths of the chromosomes in a cell. Individual characteristics by the assemblage of genes. There is a 'triggering' on and off system which determines which genes are operative at any particular time. It is all the more remarkable, therefore, that the only action they have, to achieve what they do, is to control the selection of amino acids and consequent build-up into proteins. All the rest follows.

We distinguish between germ cells, which are involved in reproduction,

A simple representation of Deoxyribonucleic Acid (DNA). The four nucleotide bases—thymine, guanine, cytosine, and adenine—always pair thymine–adenine and cytosine–guanine, and it is to be understood that the phosphate–sugar (Ph–S) chains are spirals.

Nucleotide bases:

Thymine

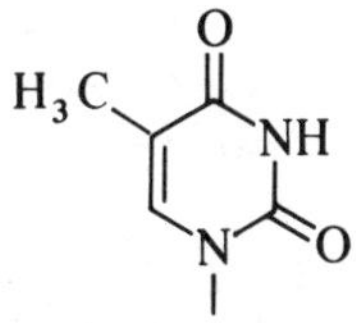

Guanine

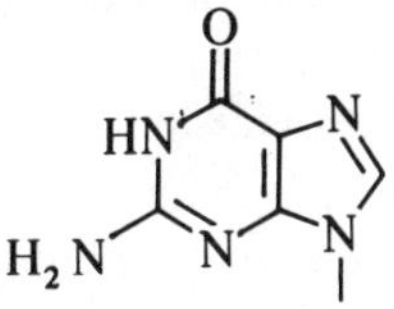

Cytosine

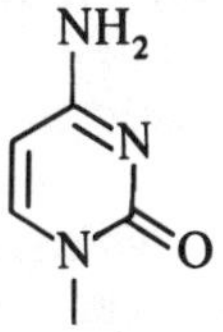

Adenine

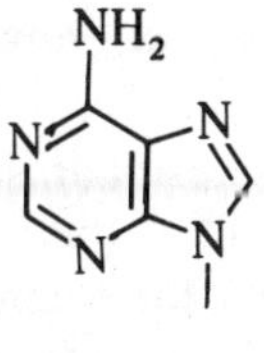

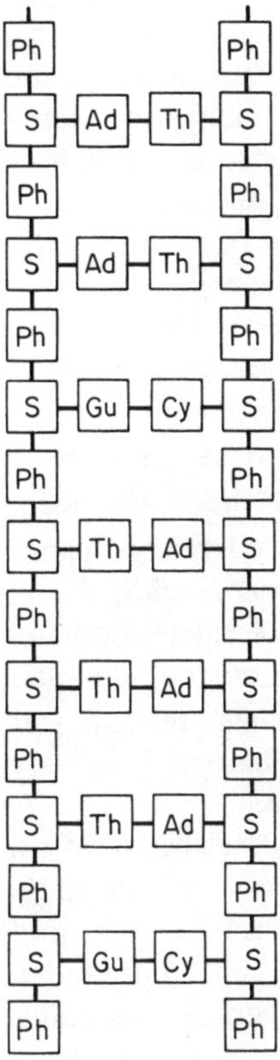

and somatic cells, which are concerned with growth and replacement. In the division of germ cells there is an interchange of some of the genes of chromosomes that pair off homologously, that is, two chromosomes of similar character but one originating with the father and the other with the mother. This process is known as meiosis. In the division of somatic cells there is simply a duplication of characteristics and the genetic information is transmitted intact. In neither case, in normal circumstances, is the hereditary information interfered with, and only in the case of meiosis is it redistributed.

A mutagen is something that does interfere[56] but its action must be clearly distinguished from that of spontaneous mutation, which can also occur, and indeed without which life would not have advanced on this planet in the way it has. So a mutagenic substance may be defined as something which increases the frequency, and adversely affects the character, of change in genetic material: in the number and structure of the chromosomes and in the composition of genes. Mutations in germ cells prior to or during the reproductive period can be transmitted to later generations, resulting in reproductive defects. (In somatic cells they may lead to carcinogenicity or teratogenicity.) It may alter a gene so that it contains a wrong code, or it may cause a chromosome to gain or lose a gene.

Because of their ease of mutation, microorganisms are used for screening, but some highly sensitive naturally occurring bacteria have been found to react in a manner that is not relevant to man and these have been excluded from screening tests. On the other hand, considerable work has gone into developing the most suitable strains of sensitive bacteria. However, no one test has been found to provide an unambiguous answer and a battery of them has been proposed,[62] some *in vitro* and some *in vivo*. The preferred microorganisms for *in vitro* studies of gene mutation are salmonella and *E. coli*, the two being complementary in response, but there are other useful test organisms. Positive controls, that is, controls in which a known mutagen is present, are essential, in addition to the normal control in which the test substance is absent. For *in vitro* chromosome aberration tests, human lymphocytes are cultured at multidose levels with the test substance.

Reference 62 describes a host-mediated *in vivo* assay for gene mutation, that is, an assay in which the experimental cell, which may be either microbial or a lymphocyte, is implanted in a host animal—usually a mouse, which is fed the substance under test. At the end of the experiment the implant is removed for examination. This test, however, is now losing favour.

For *in vivo* chromosal aberration tests Chinese hamsters or rats—and less frequently mice—are used as test animals, and at the end of the experiment bone marrow and spermatocytes are removed for examination.

Perhaps more so than in other tests, everything turns on the knowledge and expertise of the operators in organizing and carrying out the tests, and in recognizing cell defects or amino acid miscodings that may have been introduced.

One other test may be included. It is known as the dominant lethal, and it is a measure of foetal loss due to a mutagen. In it mature male rats are dosed with the test substance and then mated each week for a period of 8 weeks to small groups of females. Controls are run at the same time. At a specified point after mating, the females are killed and the number of dead implants relative to the total number recorded. Substances are suspect if there is a statistically significant increase of dead implants relative to the controls.

A teratogen is a substance that produces abnormalities in a developing embryo. The most infamous example is that of thalidomide. (The effects must not be confused with those of mutagens which produce, for example, mongols.) The main problem here has been to identify an animal species that permits one to extrapolate reasonably to human response. One might well have expected primates to be the most useful but this is not the case. Indeed a study of the effects of known teratogens on a number of species has led to the recommendation that one rodent species—rat, mouse, or hamster—and the non-rodent be used. Examination for teratogenic effects is usually carried out as part of the subchronic toxicity programme to be described later, but tests directed specifically to teratogenicity may be required. In such cases the substance is administered to the female, usually after mating but sometimes before, and the offspring are removed by Caesarian section before normal parturition is due, in order to recover all the products of conception. If it is considered advisable, the other offspring are reared to maturity for continued study.

A carcinogen is a substance that produces cancer in a test organism, and tests for cancer are usually carried out with rats and/or mice. Insofar as there can be differences in sex response and in strain response (particularly with respect to spontaneous tumour response) it follows that specific thought must be given to the selection of animals when designing an experiment. Furthermore, cancer is normally a delayed aberration effect and tests need to be continued over the major part of the animals' lifetime. So they are usually fitted into the pattern of long-term chronic toxicity programmes. Nevertheless, here again it could be that carcinogenicity is the sole concern of the investigation. In such a case it is advantageous to use specific-pathogen-free animals since their life expectation under normal dietary conditions is that much longer.

A comprehensive comparison of animal species response to both teratogens and carcinogens is given in one of the source references 63.

Subchronic Toxicity Tests

In this section, and in the one that follows, we are concerned with what used to be called subacute toxicity, distinguished from acute toxicity by the fact that the substance did not yield immediate toxic symptoms, but only after cumulative ingestion. This simple descriptive distinction served during the early years of investigation, but knowledge has now grown to a point that permits more exact definition. It has been a progressive situation in which the kinds of tests that were devised—short term and long-term—foreshadowed the division that was to come. Originally the so-called short-term tests did not extend beyond 90 days for rodents, or one tenth of life expectation for non-rodents, but multigeneration testing may now push the period well beyond these points.

102

Currently the aims of the tests are:

1. to determine the effects of protracted feeding of a test substance to animals at various dose levels covering a non-toxic/toxic range;
2. to examine the consequential effects on reproduction, usually over several generations, and including the possibility of abnormality in the offspring:
3. to collate and evaluate the data relative to the possible risk to humans.

For these purposes the tests may extend over a year or more in order to collect sufficient data to characterize and assess the physiological and pathological consequences of continued ingestion of the substance at something lower than the lethal level. The LD_{50} value may be used as a guide to dosing levels, or it may be thought better to run a short (3–4 weeks) test with small groups of animals at a number of levels. In this the lowest level would be somewhat higher than the intended level of addition to food, but expectedly having no toxic effect. The highest level would need to produce a toxic effect. In such a pre-run the animals would finally be killed off for post-mortem examination, as a guide for effects to be looked for in a more rigorous 90-day test that provides the framework for subchronic toxicity investigations.

As has been already indicated, the 90-day test may be so organized as to provide investigation of possible reproductive and teratogenetic defects. Specified procedures are necessary to maintain good husbandry, and the animals must be selected to limit variability and maximize response. In a typical test, groups of 20 rodents of each sex for each dose level, and of 3 or 4 non-rodents (each with duplicate control groups) would be used. The animals are weanlings, and preferably litter mates for test and control. The non-rodents are there more for qualitative confirmation of the trend of the experiment, the sample being too small for statistical evaluation. Just what measurements and examinations are to be carried out will depend on the experience and prior knowledge of the operators, and there may be limited objectives. In totality they will cover:

Physical examination:

Checks for appearance, morbidity, mortality.
Examination for toxic signs or deviant activity, posture or behaviour.
Records of food consumption and body weight.
Tests for neurological response and opthalmologic changes.
Functional tests—cardiovascular, hepatic, renal, respiratory.

Haematological examination:

Haemoglobin, haematocrit, red/white cell counts, total white cell and differential count, platelets, reticulocytes, prothrombin, clotting times.

Biochemical evaluation:

Blood glucose, urea nitrogen, creatinene.
Serum albumin/globulin ratio.
Serum lipids (cholesterol, glycerides, fatty acids).
Serum electrolytes and osmolarity.
Serum enzymes (transaminases, phosphatases).
Functional tests (bromsulphthalein and urea clearance in large animals).

Faecal analyses:

Occult blood.
Moisture content.

Post-mortem examination:

Gross necropsy.
Organ weights.
Histopathology.

Urine analyses:

Sugars, urea nitrogen, bilirubin
Protein
Ketones
Enzymes
Trace minerals, metabolites etc.

Now it is unlikely that all readers will know what all the tests listed above involve. Nor is it important that they should. The list is included to underline the potential exhaustiveness of safety evaluation at this stage. It also illustrates the application of the disciplinary exercises set out earlier on page 97 of this chapter.

The tests, or a selection of them, may be embodied in a multigeneration experiment such as that set out in Figure 1. This is designed to study the effects of the substance on fertility and on the normality of the offspring; and also possible carry-through of other effects from generation to generation.

It could be that a clear indication of the conditions under which a substance could be judged safe might be reached at this stage, except that in certain circumstances, such as the addition of substances to staple foods, tests to establish freedom from carcinogenicity are mandatory.

Chronic Toxicity Tests

A decision whether or not to proceed to a full span of chronic toxicity tests will depend on expert assessment of the results and data assembled at this point. There would be rejection of the substance if the overall effects of maximum likely human consumption were judged to be socially unacceptable. On the other hand, if they were found acceptable, if the human 'dosage' level was reasonably low, if the genetic toxicity tests were favourable, and if there were unassailable arguments for the absence of carcinogenetic activity, then a recommendation to approve the substance could be made. Otherwise, if there were doubts on any one of the four conditions listed here, then chronic toxicity tests would be indicated.

Basically, such tests consist of long-term experiments which have for

Food Additive Multigeneration Breeding Study

Summarized Programme for test and control groups

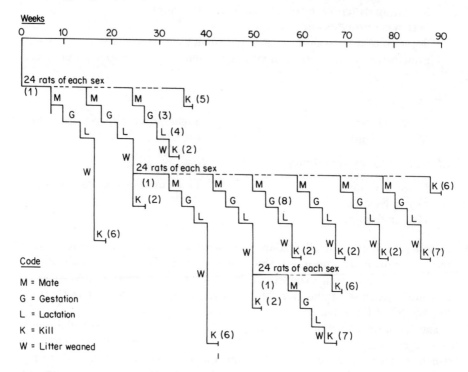

Code

M = Mate
G = Gestation
L = Lactation
K = Kill
W = Litter weaned

Instructions

(1) Body weights, food intake, water intake.
(2) Gross autopsy.
(3) Kill 50% pregnant rats on day 20: examine foetuses.
(4) Collect milk: analyse for metabolites.
(5) Blood analysis: gross autopsy.
(6) Urine and blood analysis: organ weights and tissue tests: gross autopsy.
(7) As (6) but with histological examination.
(8) Behaviour studies.

Figure 1. *Food Additive Multigeneraton Breeding Study.* (*Summarized programme for test and control groups.*)

their aim to identify and characterize toxic effects that become evident only after prolonged exposure to a test substance, though they can also duplicate to any required extent subchronic tests. Since they are spread over the lifetime of the animal, it is best that the animal has a short life span if the tests are not to be unduly protracted. This means using rats and mice, but a vast experience has been built up over the years on, for example, the choice of strain (with respect to health and variation of response with increasing age), disease resistance, and probability of premature death (this to avoid undue loss of animals over the longer period of the test).

It is important that any experiment is very carefully planned for once it is started, the conditions cannot be altered without destroying the validity of the results. If the design is found to be faulty the experiment has to be abandoned and that is wasteful of time and money. It may occasionally be considered useful to undertake periodic slaughtering of small groups of animals for intermediate autopsy, but this is not often done. However, whether or not this is done will determine the number of animals required but there must be a sufficient number at the end to allow statistical treatment of the data. The aim is to so design the experiment that it follows a path leading to the most positive conclusion.

Each experiment has its own protocol and the number of animals required will depend on this. As a rough guide, 40–60 animals will be required for each dose level test to ensure an adequate number of survivors after 2 years, and up to 8 non-rodents. Controls will contain double the number of animals since there is usually only one control group for all the test levels. These levels are best chosen on the basis of the subchronic test results, the highest dose level being one that has produced a toxic effect without a significant increase in mortality. The experiment may be carried through to a second generation.

The normal period of the experiment is not less than 2 years. Should it be decided to have interim sacrifices these would take place at 6, 12, and 18 months, and the animals would receive the same clinical, biochemical, and pathological examinations as at full term. These are not mandatory. There is a more selective protocol than for subchronic testing, with an emphasis on post-mortem pathological examination, with particular reference to carcinogenesis. Pathologists therefore play a correspondingly larger part in the summing up and subsequent judgement.

To summarize then, modern safety testing is assuming the shape of a sequential programme in which many disciplines are involved. It has led to the concept of a decision-making tree whereby acutely toxic substances are eliminated at the first stage, and the conditions under which other substances could be accepted in subsequent stages. It is based on the concept that no constituent of food, additive or otherwise, is safe for all levels or conditions of ingestion, and it is concerned to establish safe levels for additives. In all cases a judgement is required but it is more easily reached in some cases than in others. It is based on an assessment of risk. The aim of the tests, taken together, is to reveal all relevant factors and take them into account in a manner that permits a valid judgement to be made.

APPENDIX A

The Toxicant Risks of Natural Food

There are two comprehensive texts on the toxicity of natural foods[64,65] for those who wish to know more of the subject than is dealt with here. Both publications consist of contributions by experts on the various categories of toxic substances. In addition there are a number of more recent reviews, most of which have made ample use of the texts. This appendix, in turn, has relied very much on the reviews. Some of the examples quoted are of foods not normally consumed in developed countries, but current concern so far as food is concerned is perhaps more with underdeveloped countries. Furthermore, in view of the world-wide search for new plant food sources, knowledge of this kind can become totally relevant. The primary purpose here, however, is to ensure the safety of food additives; there is a somewhat cavalier attitude towards the presence of toxic substances in food. Indeed most people eat such food unaware of the inherent risks, mainly because their cooking and eating habits do not lead to excessive levels of the toxicant in the body and if, by some misjudgement, there should be excess, the cause of the consequent ailment is often looked for elsewhere. This leads to the general statement that a toxic substance presents a risk, normally in one of three conditions:

A detoxification procedure has not been carried out.

The food is eaten in excess amounts.

The food is eaten by people who react abnormally.

Toxic substances can be dealt with conveniently under the following groupings:

Constituents of natural food products.

Contaminants of natural food products of microbiological origin.

Contaminants of natural food products of non-microbiological origin.

Constituents of Natural Food Products

Oxalates. A surprising number of common foods contain a combined form of oxalic acid, usually acid potassium oxalate. Among them are rhubarb, spinach, celery, beetroot, parsley, almond, and tea. Normally there is sufficient calcium in other food items to immobilize the acid as the calcium salt, but there have been cases of poisoning due to excessive consumption. The quantity in tea, for example, is low, the risk coming from the amount drunk.

Acid potassium oxalate

$$
\begin{array}{c}
\text{COOH} \\
| \\
\text{COOK}
\end{array}
$$

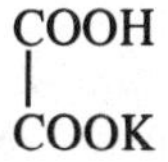

Cyanogens. A number of plants contain glycosides that can break down and release cyanic acid into the system. This then inhibits the action of cytochrome oxidase in the respiratory cycle. The highest levels of the glycoside have been found in cassava (manioc), Lima bean and sorghum millet. Other plants that contain it are the kidney bean, garden pea, sweet potato, Indian gram, and almond. The glycoside has been named linamarin.

Linamarin (phaseolunatin)

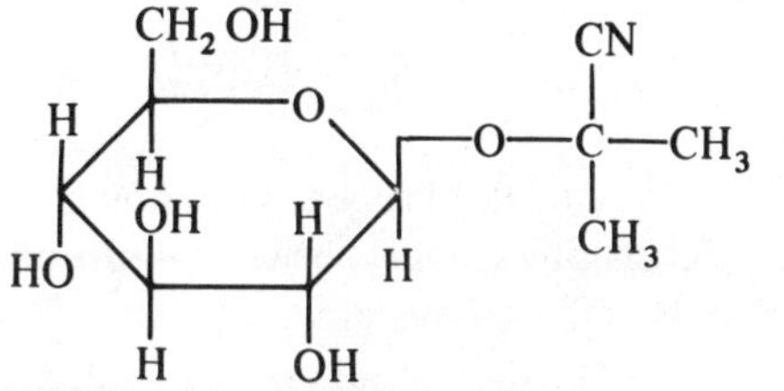

Improperly prepared cassava has been associated with two diseases—amblyopia (blindness) and ataxic neuropathy (a degenerative disease)—in West Africa, particularly Nigeria. Those native communities aware of the danger avoid it by means of a soaking and fermentation process. Attempts are being made to introduce cereal and legume crops to replace cassava, but there are difficulties to be overcome.[10] There is also a long-term programme to produce a cassava plant free of the glycoside.

Lima beans were responsible for outbreaks of poisoning in Europe in the early part of this century. Nowadays selection is made on the basis of low glycoside content and this is further reduced by a soaking and washing process.

Safrole. This compound, a mild carcinogen, is a substituted phenol. It is present in the potato as well as in a number of spices. It is closely related

Safrole

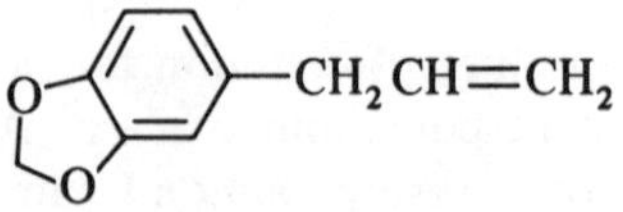

to eugenol and vanillin. It was popular as a flavour additive to beer in the U.S. but is no longer permitted.

Goitrogens. The common cause of goitre is a shortage of iodine in the diet, but it is not the only cause. Some plants contain thioglycosides that break down and release an agent that interferes with the metabolism of iodine to produce a goitre. Two such agents have been identified—allyl isothiocyanate and 5-vinyloxazolidine-2-thione. Thioglycosides responsible for one or other of them have been found in the soya bean and in most members of the Brassica family—cabbage, turnip, cauliflower, kale, Brussels sprouts, broccoli. The level is low in the Brassicas, and cooking eliminates any risk, but there have been reports of goitre in rural Indian communities due to an excessive consumption, and of an interesting case in Tasmania[66] where children were affected by milk from cows fed continuously on kale.

Allyl isothiocyanate   S-5-Vinyloxazolidine-2-thione

$CH_2=CHCH_2N=C=S$

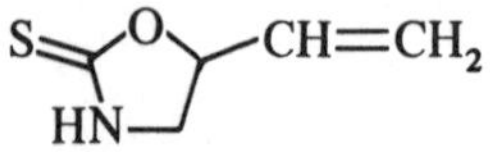

Lathyrogens. Two kinds of lathyrogen are known. One—osteolathyrogen —causes skeletal deformities: the other—neurolathyrogen—can cause paralysis of the central nervous system and of the lower limbs. The first, so far as is known, affects only animals. The other affects humans and provides support for the argument that it is not necessarily the presence *per se* of a toxic material but the level at which it is present that creates a risk.

In parts of India wheat and chickling vetch (*Lathyrus sativus*) are cultivated and mixed off for consumption. In normal times wheat provides the major part of the mixture, but in drought conditions the vetch survives better and the proportion of it in the mixture is increased. This has now been explicitly related to rises in incidence of lathyrism, particularly among young adult males, when the proportion of vetch increases above a threshold value. Lathyrism used to be common in Mediterranean countries, and still breaks out intermittently in India and Eritrea, presumably because of ignorance of the cause.

There are two suspected causative agents, β-N-oxalyl-α,β-diaminopropionic acid and α, β-diaminopropionic acid, but the point has been made[67] that if

β-N-Oxalyl-α,β-diaminopropionic acid

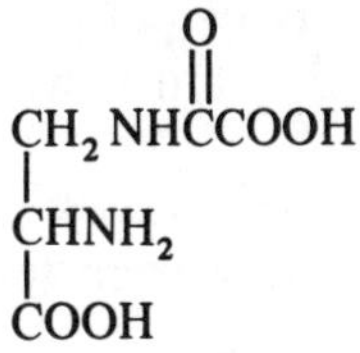

$$CH_2NHCCOOH$$
$$\overset{O}{\overset{\|}{}}$$

CH₂NHCCOOH
|
CHNH₂
|
COOH

α,β-Diaminopropionic acid

CH₂NH₂
|
CHNH₂
|
COOH

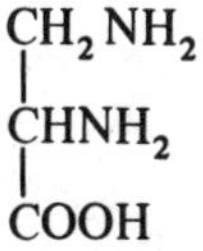

this is so, a simple detoxification procedure should be possible and an otherwise valuable source of food made safe.

Cycasin. Seeds of the cycad plant contain cycasin, a glycoside. This is susceptible to bacterial attack when it breaks down and produces a potent carcinogen, methylazoxymethanol (MAM). The seeds are cooked and eaten by the indigenous population of a group of Pacific islands that includes Guam; but only if they are well soaked and washed before cooking are ill effects to be avoided.

Cycasin

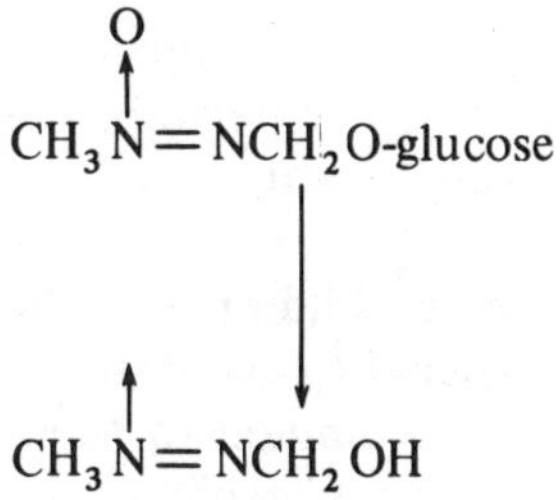

$$CH_3 \overset{O}{\underset{\uparrow}{N}} = NCH_2O\text{-glucose}$$

$$CH_3 \overset{\uparrow}{N} = NCH_2OH$$

Methylazoxymethanol (MAM)

Solanine. This substance is an alkaloidal glycoside present in a number of plants of which the potato is the most important. It is a cholinesterase inhibitor, pharmacologically similar to nerve gas,[7] interfering with the transmission of nerve impulses. The concentration in the potato increases when the tuber is exposed to light and turns green, and even more so when

Solanidine (Solanine, referred to in the text, is a trisaccharide derivative of solanidine, of the form rhamnose-galactose-glucose-solanidine.)

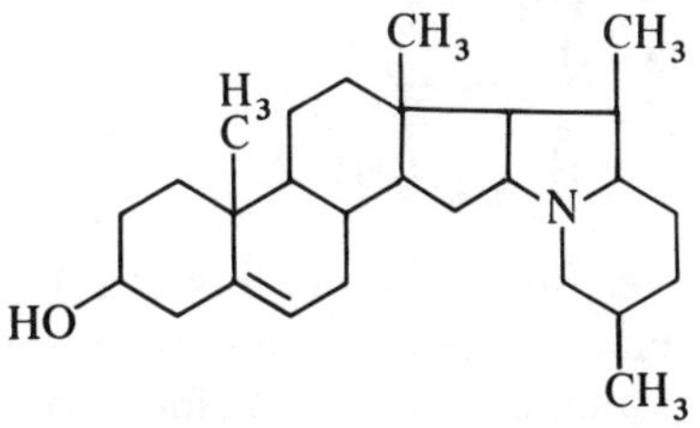

110

sprouting takes place. The clearest evidence of poisoning has come from eating cooked sprouting potatoes.[66] Recently a new variety of potato was developed with improved chipping and browning properties, but it had to be rejected because of its high level of solanine.[8]

Pyrrolizidine. Some species of groundsel (*Senecio*) are occasionally cooked and eaten by Bantu tribes in South Africa. They have been found to contain the carcinogenetic alkaloid, pyrrolizidine.[68]

Pyrrolizidine

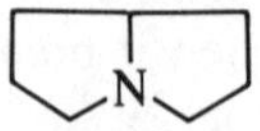

Trypsin inhibitors. These are proteinaceous materials that interfere with the process of food digestion, trypsin being one of the pancreatic enzymes involved. They are present in the groundnut, soya bean, navy bean and Lima bean. They must be inactivated by steaming or cooking.

Haemagglutinins. These substances are also proteinaceous and cause red blood cells to clump together, so impairing their action. They are constituents of the soya bean, Guatemalan red bean, Indian red gram, and Philippine mung bean. Soaking in water, followed by cooking, is necessary to inactivate them.

Coeliac disease. Some young children are allergic to wheat gluten, but there is no solution to this, except to avoid it.

Favism. This is an affliction common to those people whose red blood cells are deficient in glucose-6-phosphate dehydrogenase (an enzyme involved in hydrogen transport). It is confined to Caucasian-type inhabitants of countries in the Mediterranean basin, or who originated there. It is a haemolytic anaemia brought on by eating broad beans (*Vicia Fava*) and the causative agent is thought to be a glucose-containing nucleotide named vicine.

Vicine

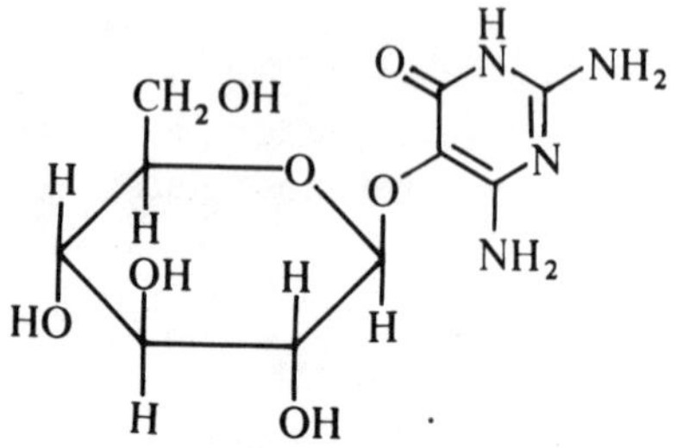

Amines. Certain amines and some cheeses affect people who are taking antidepressant drugs. Plants which contain such amines are the banana, tomato, avocado. The amines are adrenaline, noradrenaline, dopamine,

Adrenaline

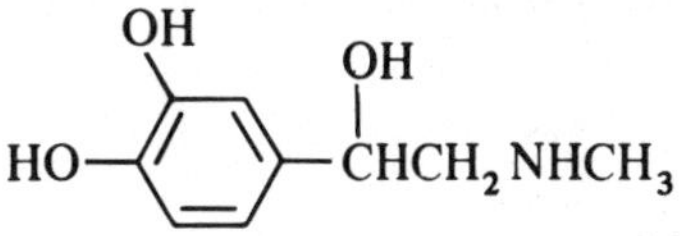

Noradrenaline

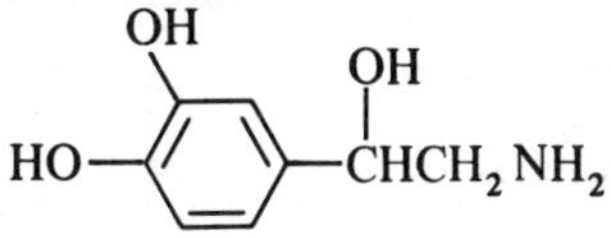

Dopamine

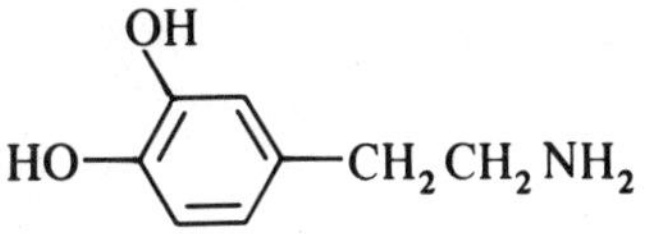

Tyramine

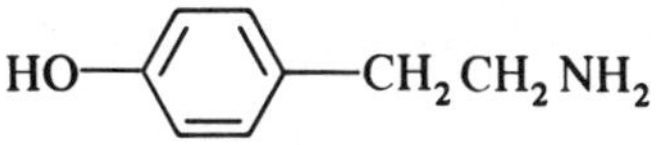

Histamine

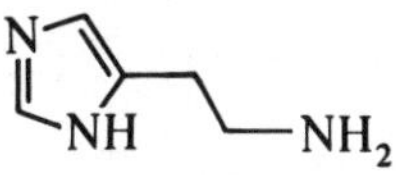

tyramine, histamine, and tryptamine. These elevate blood pressure but in normal circumstances they are detoxified by a monoamine oxidase. The drugs inhibit the enzyme.

Serotonin
(5-Hydroxytryptamine)

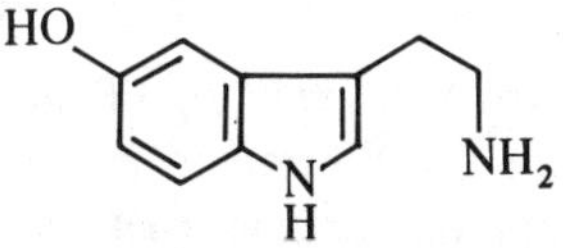

Plantains contain another amine, serotonin, which thought to be responsible for a heart condition among African tribes. To offset this, attempts are being made to introduce cereals and legumes to reduce dependence on the plantains.

Hypoglycins. Ackee fruit, commonly eaten in the West Indies and South America, contains unusual amino acids named hypoglycins because they depress the blood sugar level and cause hypoglycaemia.

Hypoglycin A

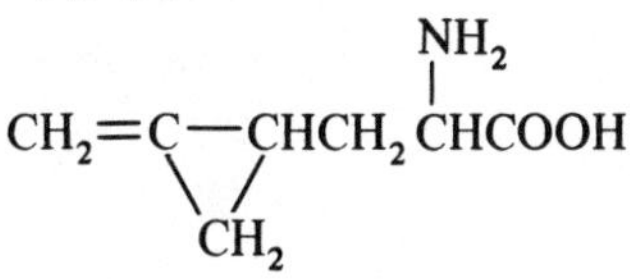

Hypoglycin B

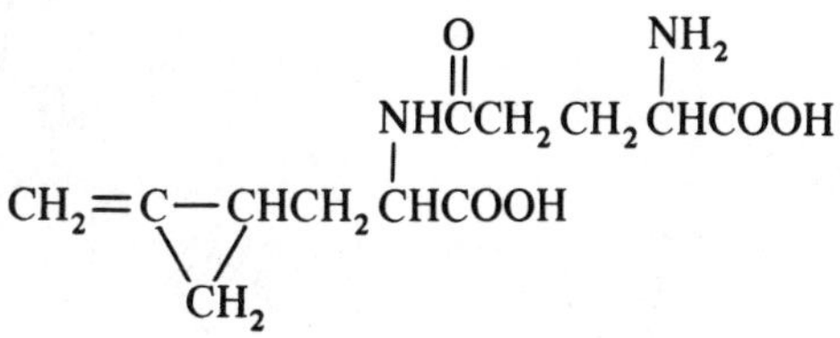

Djenkolic acid. The Djenkol bean, a popular source of food in parts of Indonesia, contains djenkolic acid which can cause oliguria, albuminuria, and renal colic.

Djenkolic acid

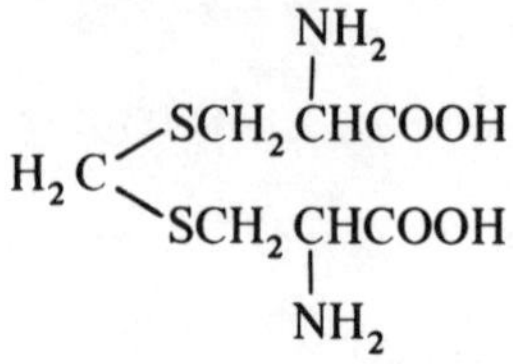

$$H_2C \underset{\displaystyle SCH_2 \underset{\displaystyle NH_2}{\overset{\displaystyle NH_2}{CHCOOH}}}{\overset{\displaystyle SCH_2 \overset{\displaystyle NH_2}{CHCOOH}}{<}}$$

3,4-Benzpyrene. This, and other carcinogenic polynuclear aromatic hydrocarbons have been identified in a number of vegetables,[72] as products of biosynthesis.

3,4-Benzpyrene

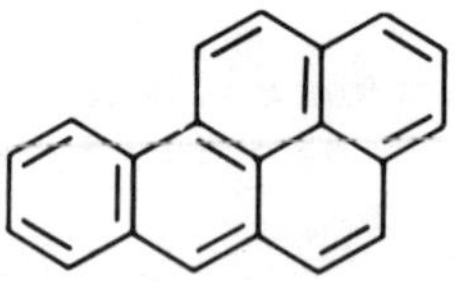

Microbiological Contaminants of natural Food Products

Aflatoxin. This is a toxin of major significance in world food supplies, though food scientists were not alerted to it by food contamination, but by an outbreak of disease among turkeys that led to high mortality. It was traced back to the use of Brazilian groundnuts in the feedstock, and from that to heavy contamination of the nuts with the mould, *Aspergillus flavus.* This led to widespread recognition of contamination of many cereals and legumes of mainly Asian and African origin. It was fortunate that the unusually heavy contamination of the Brazilian nuts alerted scientists, for the aflatoxins that the mould produces are liver carcinogens. They have now been well characterized and any source can be checked, but mould

Aflatoxin B$_1$

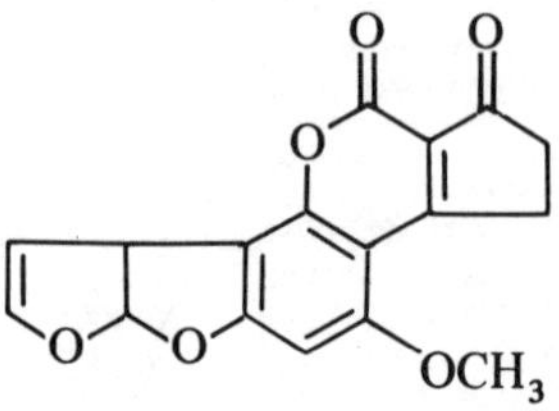

growth can be prevented only by storage of the food in cool non-humid conditions.

The problem is particularly troublesome in India where groundnut meal, from home-produced nuts, is playing an important part in India's attempts not only to become self-sufficient but also to improve the quality of the available food.[10]

Luteoskyrin and Islandicum. Improperly stored rice in Japan is susceptible to a mould growth that produces two carcinogens. The mould is *Penicillium islandicum.*

Luteoskyrin

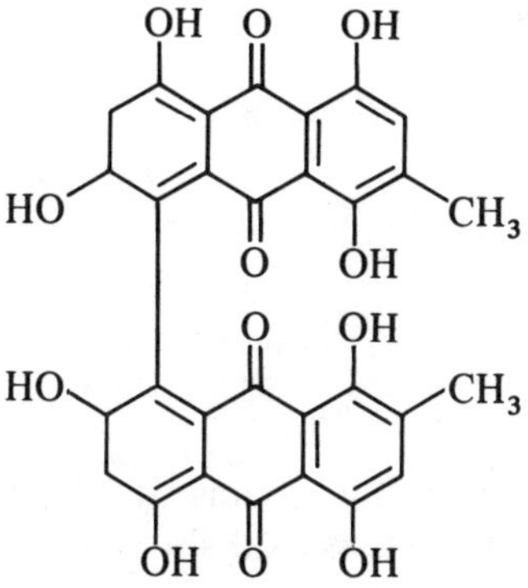

Ergot. Rye in particular, but other cereals also, are prone to attack by the mould, *Claviceps purpurea*, which contains the toxin, ergot. This is an alkaloid with two toxic effects. One causes intense pain in the extremities (known as St Anthony's fire) and possible gangrene, and the other cramp or convulsions. It was a mediaeval scourge until its cause was discovered, and there are still occasional outbreaks among rural communities, and continuing risk to simple life enthusiasts who grow their own rye.

Ergot

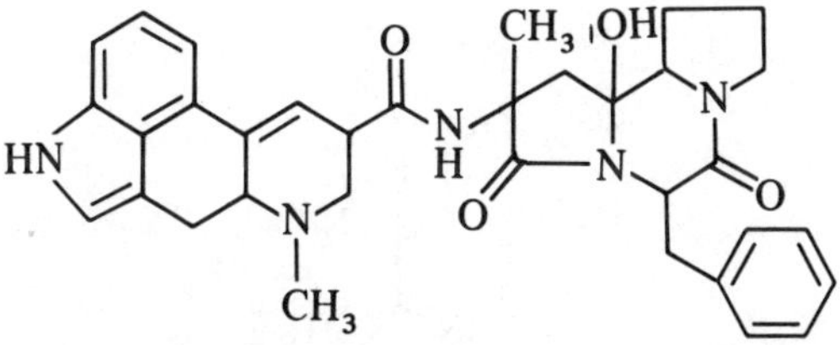

Tricothecanes. These are tetracyclic sesquiterpenes produced by *Fusarium* moulds. *Fusarium tricinctus* grows on badly stored grain and has been responsible for many deaths in Russia. *Fusarium nivali* is a

Trichothecanes

1. Toxin HT2 *ex Fusarium tricinctus*

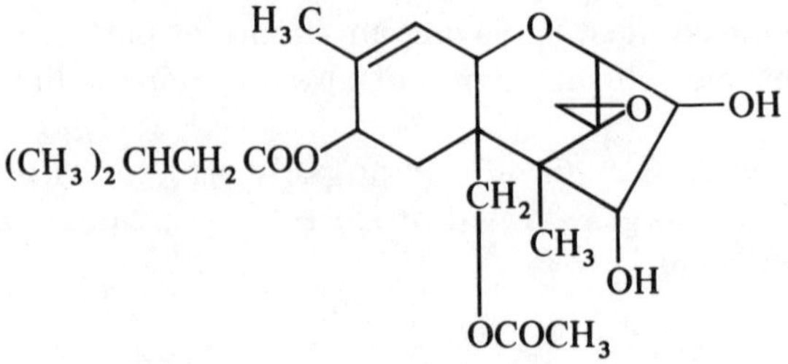

2. Nivalenol *ex Fusarium nivali*

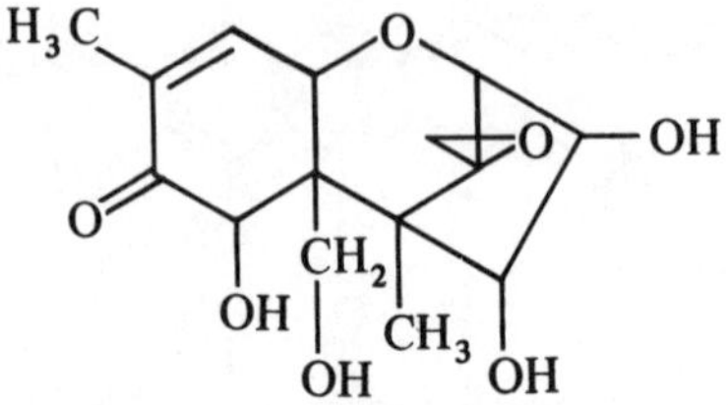

contaminant of rice and other grains in Japan and has been held responsible for a disease known as akakabi-byo.

Non-microbiological Contaminants of natural Food Products

Saxitoxin. The hazard of saxitoxin was relatively unknown in the U.K. 10 years ago, but not so now. Shellfish, such as mussels, clams, and scallops become toxic when they eat the dinoflagellate, *Gonyaulax catenella*, or *Gonyaulax tamarensis*. This proliferates occasionally in coastal waters, when it gives rise to, and can be detected by a 'red tide' which turns luminescent at night. The shellfish are immune to the toxin, but they cannot metabolize it, nor is it inactivated when the shellfish are cooked. It is paralytic in action.

Saxitoxin

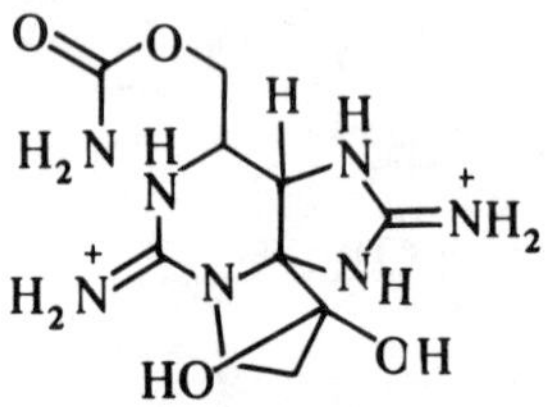

Tetradotoxin. This toxin is to be found in either the ovaries or testes of the pufferfish, which should be removed before the fish is cooked. This does not always happen. It affects respiration and has been responsible for many deaths in Japan.

Tetradotoxin

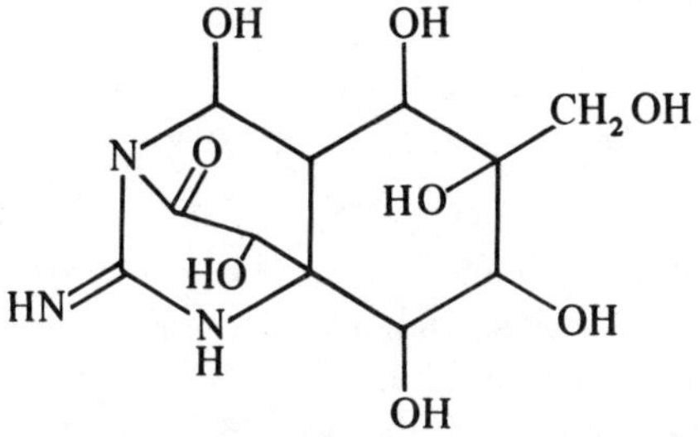

Food Additives Compilations

It is necessary, if effective use is to be made of the systematic work carried out on food additives, that lists should be compiled of substances permitted or not permitted, without or with conditions of use, in this or that country. Without such compilations there can be no ready assessment of the situation as it affects one's interests or requirements. Yet, as we shall see, there is more than one way of doing this, and the titles of those that have appeared reveal little of the variety of treatment. In this appendix, therefore, comparison is made of five useful publications that have appeared. Reference to some of them has already appeared in the main text.

Chemicals used in Food Processing

This publication is of both factual and historic interest. It was prepared by the Food Technology Subcommittee of the National Academy of Sciences—National Research Council in the U.S., and published in 1965. It was compiled from information submitted by manufacturers, and supplemented by information on definitions and standards from official sources.

It listed all the chemicals for which the committee has found authentic evidence of use and, in so doing, revealed the size of the problem to be tackled in establishing control of them, for listing does not imply approval of any item in the list. Nevertheless, insofar as many of the substances have since been approved, the compilation has not lost significance, particularly for its ancillary information.

It concerns itself only with intentional additives, that is, those added with a specific effect in mind, and not with those that might be there adventitiously, due to pesticidal treatment of a food ingredient, or to the use of a packaging material. It lists the additives in groups as follows:

Preservatives
Antioxidants
Sequestrants

Surface-active agents
Stabilizers and thickeners
Bleaching agents, maturing agents, and starch modifiers
Buffers, acids, and alkalies
Food colours
Non-nutrient and special dietary sweeteners
Nutrient supplements
Flavouring agents

    A. synthetic
    B. spices, herbs, essential oils, and plant extractives
Miscellaneous

    yeast foods, firming agents, texturizers, binders, anticaking agents, enzymes

Today the term emulsifier is preferred to surface-active agent, and not all countries, or compilers, consider nutrient supplements to be additives, though that is what they are in fact. Starch modifiers are still a matter of discussion. Flavours are dealt with more comprehensively than in any other compilation, due no doubt to the fact that they were compiled prior to any intensive legislative control. They are divided into synthetic and naturally occurring substances, but the division is a little misleading, for many of those listed as synthetic have been identified also as components of natural flavours. This raises an interesting point in passing, for some authorities, the Japanese and the Germans for example, distinguish between a natural substance and a synthetic copy of it when considering permission to use. However, there can be no doubt that the section on flavours provides a useful compendium to sparser accounts given elsewhere.

The book predates the concept of Acceptable Daily Intake and gives average maximum levels of addition instead, a figure that takes less account of the amount of food likely to be ingested.

Handbook of Food Additives

This a discursive type of book, in two parts, edited by T. E. Furia and published by C. R. C. Press in 1972. In Part 1 each group of additives is discussed by a recognised expert, the aim being to inform the reader of the reasons for and purposes of the various additives, and to indicate where possible the mechanisms whereby they achieve their respective aims. This may well be the more important part. Part 2 deals with the regulatory control of additives, but we have seen from the main text that such things are in a state of flux and, as time recedes, this may become little more than of historic interest.

Food Additives—Description, Functions, and U.K. Legislation

This was compiled by N. R. Jones and D. W. Flowerdew and first published in 1976 by the BFMIRA. Unlike the previous publication it has been issued in loose-leaf form to permit the information to be updated, but it is concerned only with activities in the U.K.

Its purpose is set out in the Introduction:

'This guide is intended to enable a general idea of the restrictions on the use of any additive to be obtained without reference to the various documents that set out the rules in full. At the same time references are made to the various Statutory Instruments involved with any particular additive so that the precise conditions under which it can be used and the permitted levels can be found.'

There is little guidance on flavours.

Index to Food Additives evaluated by the Joint FAO/WHO Expert Committee

This was compiled by C. F. King and published in 1977 by the BFMIRA with the subsidiary title—Food Legislative Surveys No. 2—unusually so insofar as FAO/WHO evaluations have no legislative authority unless given it by individual countries.

The FAO/WHO publishes all its findings in the form of either reports or monographs, and this publication is primarily a guide to original sources. It lists all the additives that have been evaluated, identifying the function of each and the ADI where this has been established, though for any qualification to this one must refer back, and this holds also for toxicological evaluation, technological efficiency, and specification. Insofar as the original sources group additives according as they are generally or tentatively approved (A), awaiting judgement (B), or either disapproved or severely restricted in use (C), it would have helped if this simple scoring had been included.

Substances are not grouped functionally but listed alphabetically. One can see at a glance therefore if any substance has more than one additive function.

Food Additive Tables

This is the most ambitious of the compilations. It is the work of the Food Law Research Centre, Institute of European Studies, University of Brussels. It is edited by E. J. Bigwood and others and first published by

Elsevier Scientific Publishing Company in 1975. It is on loose-leaf form and covers operations in the following 20 countries:

Austria, Belgium, Denmark, Finland, France, West Germany, Eire, Italy, Luxembourg, Holland, Norway, Portugal, Spain, Sweden, Switzerland, the U.K., Canada, Israel, Japan, and the U.S.

It has called for considerable ingenuity in devising a system that permits cross-referencing. The system is based, not on classes of additives, but on the kinds of foods to which they are added, and 15 groups have been selected as follows:

1. Cereal products.
2. Sugars, honey, syrups, jams, marmalades, jellies, and certain spreads.
3. Nuts and related products.
4. Potatoes and related products.
5. Vegetables, legumes, mushrooms.
6. Fruits and related products.
7. Meat, poultry, and related products.
8. Fish, shellfish, and related products.
9. Milk, milk products, and related products such as cheese.
10. Eggs (domestic birds) and related products.
11. Fats and oils, butter, and margarine.
12. Beverages and drinks.
13. Confectioneries, including chocolate and related products.
14. Seasonings, condiments, and spices.
15. Mixed products such as ready-prepared dishes.

The editors agree that the groupings are somewhat artificial, but claim that it is the most suitable for the system, which works through a series of tables, each table dealing with a subgroup of foods. Thus the first group of foods has 8 related tables, the first column of which lists the 20 countries. The other columns cover the different classes of additives. The body of each table may be thought of as a rectangle of boxes, in which each box contains a set of cyphers which have significance both by their character and by their arrangement. The meanings of the cyphers are given in supplementary lists. Thus a complete picture may be built up of the status of any additive relative to a particular kind of food in any of the 20 countries at the time the latest table was drawn up. Under the loose-leaf system no data would be more than 3 months out of date. However, in practice, these aims have not been achieved.

Source References

1. Leopold, A. C. and Ardrey, R., Toxic substances in plants and the food habits of early man, *Science*, **176**, 512 (1972).
2. Bernal, J. D., *Science in History*, C. A. Wallis & Co., (1969).
3. *Conservation of Plant Genetic Resources* (Ed. J. G. Hughes), *British Association for the Advancement of Science*, University of Aston in Birmingham (1978).
4. *Guidelines for developing an effective National Food Control System, Historical Aspects*, FAO/WHO, (1976).
5. Taylor, R. J., Micronutrients, *Unilever Educational Booklet*, No. 9 (1978).
6. Fisher, P. and Bender, A., *The Value of Food*, Oxford University Press (1970).
7. Panel on Chemicals and Health of the President's Scientific Advisory Committee, National Science Foundation, U.S.A. (1973).
8. Naturally occurring toxicants in food: Expert panel of the Institute of Food Technologists, *J. Food Sci.*, **40**, 215 (1975).
9. *Dietary Goals for the United States: Select Committee on Nutrition and Human Needs*, U.S. Senate, U.S. Government Printing Office (1977).
10. Orr, E., *The Use of Protein-Rich Foods for the Relief of Malnutrition*, Tropical Products Institute (1972).
11. Higgins, M., Soy products in national and international food programs, *J. Amer. Oil Chem. Soc.*, **51**, 143A (1974).
12. Goldenburg, N., *Colours—do we need them? Why Additives?*, Forbes Publications, London (1977), p. 22.
13. O'Keefe, J., Food additives—essential tools for food production and distribution, *Food in Canada* (April 1975), p. 61.
14. Hollingsworth, D., *Nutritive Additives: Why Additives?* Forbes Publication, London (1977), p. 32.
15. Kent-Jones, D. W., Modern food and food additives, *Chem. and Ind.*, 1275 (November 1971).
16. Gurr, M. I. and James, A. T., *Lipid Biochemistry*, Chapman and Hall (1971).
17. Hampson, G. C. and Hudson, B. J. F., *Chemistry and Technology of Edible Oils and Fats* (Eds. Devine, J. and Williams, P. N.), Pergamon Press (1960).
18. S.I. 1978, No. 105, *The Antioxidants in Food Regulations*, H.M.S.O. London (1978).
19. An index to food additives evaluated by the Joint FAO/WHO Expert Committee on Food Additives, *Food Legislative Survey*, No 2, BFMIRA (1977).
20. S.I. 1975, No. 1487, *The Preservatives in Foods Regulations*, H.M.S.O. London (1975).
21. Chichester, D. F. and Tanner, F. W., *Handbook of Food Additives* (Ed. Furia, T. E.), CRC Press (1972).
22. Michaelsson, G. and Huhlin, L., *Brit. J. Dermatol.*, **88**, 525 (1975).

23. Doeglass, H. M. G., *Brit. J. Dermatol.*, **93**, 135 (1975).
24. *Report on the review of the Emulsifiers and Stabilisers in Food Regulations 1962*, MAFF, H.M.S.O. London (1970).
25. S.I. 1975, No. 1486, *The Emulsifiers and Stabilisers in Food Regulations*, H.M.S.O., London (1975).
26. S.I. 1973, No. 1340, *The Colouring Matter in Foods Regulations*, H.M.S.O., London (1973).
27. *Food Additives in Japan*, 6th edn., (1976), translation prepared by BFMIRA (1977).
28. *The Prevention of Food Adulteration Act 1954*, amended 1971, Ram Narain Lal Beni Prasad, Allahabad, India (1971).
29. Counsell, J. N., Colouring foods with carotenoids., *Flavour Industry*, **2**, 519 (1971).
30. *Chemicals used in Food Processing*, Publication No. 1274, National Academy of Sciences/National Research Council, Washington D.C. (1965).
31. *Report on the Review of Flavourings in Food*, FAC/REP/22, H.M.S.O., London (1976).
32. *Report of Further Classes of Additives*, H.M.S.O., London (1968).
33. Birch, G. G., *British Nutrition Foundation Bulletin*, No. 12 (1974), p. 23.
34. *Saccharin, the present position*, *British Nutrition Foundation Bulletin*, No. 7 (1972), p. 12.
35. Parker, K. J., *Natural high intensity sweeteners, British Nutrition Foundation Bulletin*, No. 16 (1976), p. 240.
36. *Enzymes in Food Processing* (Ed. Reed, G.), Academic Press (1975).
37. Evaluation of certain food additives: 21st Report of the Joint FAO/WHO Expert Committee on Food Additives, *WHO Technical Report Series 617*, Geneva (1978).
38. Toxicological evaluation of some enzymes, etc: (a) *WHO Food Additive Series*, No. 1 (1972); (b) *WHO Food Additive Series*, No. 6 (1975), Geneva.
39. S.I. 1963, No. 1435, *The Bread and Flour Regulations*, H.M.S.O., London (1963).
40. Knight, R. A., *Bread and Flour: Why Additives?*, Forbes Publications, London (1977), p. 36.
41. Elton, G. A. H. and Fisher, N., Flour and bread, *British Nutrition Foundation Bulletin*, No. 4 (1970), p. 17.
42. Taylor, R.J., Micronutrients, *Unilever Educational Booklet*, No. 9 (1978).
43. Federal Register, **40**, No. 103 (May 1975).
44. Taylor, R. J., Plant protein foods, *Unilever Educational Booklet*, No. 11 (1976).
45. Bender, A. E., *The fate of Vitamins in Food Processing Operations*, (Ed. Stein, M.), University of Nottingham Seminar on Vitamins, session 3 (1971).
46. S.I. 1970, No. 400, *The Labelling of Food Regulations*, H.M.S.O., (1970).
47. Coates, M. E., Nutrition and the microflora of the gastrointestinal tract, *British Nutrition Foundation Bulletin*, No. 9 (1973, p. 34.
48. Sunshine, G. A., Regulatory aspects of food additives, *Food Drug Cosmetic Law Journal*, 264 (May 1976), *31*.
49. Federal Register, **40**, No. 103 (May 1975).
50. Crampton, R. F., Cyclamates, *British Nutrition Foundation Bulletin*, No. 4 (1970), p. 14.
51. Roberts, H. R., Food additives—a study in the evaluation of safety, *Food Drug Cosmetic Law Journal*, 404, (July 1976), *31*.
52. Harkins, R. W., Food additive safety evaluation, *Food Drug Cosmetic Law Journal*, 182, (April 1977), *32*.
53. Giles, R. F., *Development of Food Legislation in the UK.*, Paper presented at the Food Quality and Safety Symposium, London, (October 1975).

54. Weedon, B. C. L., *Food Additives and Contaminants and the role of the FACC*, Paper presented at the Food Quality and Safety Symposium, London (October 1975).
55. *Memorandum on Procedure for Submissions on Food Additives and on Methods of Toxicity Testing*, H.M.S.O., London (1965).
56. *Guidelines on Mutagenicity Screening*, (REF A/C 385/14 (COMA (Chem)/ Mut/22)) Department of Health and Social Science, London, (October 1076).
57. Zimmerman, J. G., Food law—international, *Food Drug Cosmetic Law Journal*, 218 (April 1976), *31*.
58. Standards for investigation and discussion by the Food Sanitation Investigation Council of registering food additives, *Food Additives in Japan*, 4th edn. Ministry of Health and Welfare, Tokyo, 1974.
59. *Guidelines for Developing an Effective National Control System*, U.N. Environment Programme, FAO/WHO, Rome (1976).
60. *Introduction to List of Additives evaluated for their Safety-in-use*, First Series, CAC/FAL 1–1973, Codex Alimentarius Commission, FAO/WHO (1973).
61. *Procedural Manual*, 4th edn., Codex Alimentarius Commission, FAO/WHO, (1975).
62. *Proposed System for Food Safety Assessment: Food and Cosmetic Toxicology*, Vol. 16, Supplement 2, Pergamon Press (1978).
63. *Methods in Toxicology* (Ed. Paget, G. E.), Blackwell (1970).
64. *Toxicant Constituents of Plant Foodstuffs*, 2nd edn. (Ed. Liener, I. E.), Academic Press (1969).
65. *Toxicants Occurring Naturally in Foods*, National Academy of Sciences, Washington D.C. (1973).
66. Bicknell, F., *Chemicals in Food*, Faber and Faber (1960).
67. Liener, I. E., Toxic factors in protein foods, chapter in *Proteins in Human Nutrition* (Eds. Porter, J. W. G. and Rolls, B. A.), Academic Press (1973).
68. Sapeika, N., The toxicity of foods of natural origin, *Trans. Roy. Soc. Afr.*, **41**, 1 (1974).
69. *FACC Interim Report on the Review of the Colouring Matter in Food Regulations 1973*, FAC/REP/29: H.M.S.O. London (1979).
70. Haigh, R., Harmonization of legislation on foodstuffs, food additives and contaminants in the European Economic Community: Part I: Working procedures, *J. Fd. Technol.*, **13**, 255 (1978).
71. Haigh, R., Harmonization of legislation on foodstuffs, food additives and contaminants in the European Economic Community: Part II: Achievements and programme, *J. Fd. Technol.*, **13**, 491 (1978).
72. *Chemicals and Health: Report of the Panel on Chemicals and Health of the President's Science Advisory Committee* (chap 6, page 64), September 1973: Science and Technology Policy Office: National Science Foundation, USA.
73. S.I. 1974, No. 1121, *The Miscellaneous Additives in Food Regulations*. H.M.S.O. London (1974).

Index

Acids, 52
ADI (acceptable daily intake), 13, 38, 56, 90–92
Affluent society, 8, 9
Aflatoxin, 112
Aging, 12
Amines, 110
Amino acids, 5, 50, 56, 69
Ammonium phosphatides, 24
Amylase, 60
Animal laboratories, 95
Anthocyanins, 33
Anticaking agents, 50–52
  U.K. list, 51
Antioxidants, 13–19
  U.K. list, 17
Arachidonic acid, 15
Arthrobacter, 60
Ascorbic acid, 17, 70, 72
Ascorbyl palmitate, 18
Aspartame, 54
Aspergillus crysae, 60
Aspergillus flavus, 112
Aspergillus niger, 59, 60

Bacillus cereus, 59
Bacillus subtilis, 60
Baking, 12
Bases, 52
Benzoic acid, 20, 21
Biotin, 67
Bleaching agents, 72
Botulinum, 20
Bread, 12, 72
Breadmaking, 73
Buffers, 52
Butylated compounds, 18
Butylated hydroxyanisole, 16
Butylated hydroxytoluene, 16

Calcium, 12, 68
Canning, 19
Caramel, 36
Carbohydrases, 60
Carbons, double bonded, 14
Carcinogenicity, 20, 26, 55, 78, 100, 101, 112, 113
Cassava, 107
Cereals, 2
Cheese products, 24
Chemicals in food, 7, 74, 116
Chlorine dioxide, 73
Chocolate making, 24
Choline, 23
Chromosal aberration tests, 100
Chromosomes, 98, 99
Citric acid, 50
Claviceps purpura, 113
Clostridium botulinum, 20
Cobalamin, 66
Cobalt, 66, 68
Codex Alimentarius Commission, 89, 90, 92
Coeliac disease, 110
Collagen, 58
Copper, 67
Crisping agents, 53
Cro-Magnon man, 1
Cultivation, 3
Cyanogens, 107
Cyasin, 109
Cyclamate, 54, 55, 56, 78

Deficiency diseases, 4
Deficiency symptoms, 65
Deoxyribonucleic acid (DNA), 98, 99
Diglycerides, 14, 23
Dipeptide, 54
Djenkolic acid, 112

Japan, 38, 87

Lathyrogens, 108
LD_{50} value, 102
Lecithins, 22–24
Legislation, 71, 74–87, 88
  American practice, 74–81
  Eastern countries, 86–87
  EEC practice, 85–86
  U.K. practice, 81–85, 118
Lima beans, 107
Linamarin, 107
Linoleic acid, 15
Luteoskyrin, 113

Magnesium, 68
Maillard reaction, 59
Manganese, 67
Mannitol, 56
Manuring, 3
Meiosis, 99
Methanol, 21, 22
Micrococcus lysodeikticus, 60
Milk, 59
Millets, 3
Minerals, 6, 68–71
Molybdenum, 68
Monoglycerides, 14, 23
Monosaccharides, 56
Mosaic rules, 4
Mucor michei, 59
Mucor pusillus, 59
Multigeneration Breeding Study, 104
Mutagenicity testing, 96
Mutagens, 99
Mutations, 100

Natural foods
  constituents of, 107
  microbiological contaminants, 112
  non-microbiological contaminants,
    114–115
  toxicant risks, 106–115
Nicotinic acid, 70
Ninety-day test, 102
Nisin, 20
Nitrogen trichloride, 73
Nitrosoamine, 20
Nordihydroguaiaretic acid, 17, 19
Nutrition, 3–5, 10
Nutritive additives, 61–67

Oxalates, 107
Oxidation, 15
Oxidizing agents, 72

Palatability, 10
Pantothenic acid, 66
Papain, 58
Paracelsus, 5
Penicillium islandicum, 113
Pepsin, 59
Peroxidase, 59
Phenolic compounds, 18
Phosphates, 50
Phosphatides, 22
Phospholipids, 23
Phosphorus, 68
Poison, 5
Polyoxyethylene, 24
Potassium, 69
Preservatives, 19–21, 73
  basic list of, 20
Propionic acid, 21, 73
Prostaglandins, 15
Proteases, 59
Protein synthesis, 46, 57
Proteins, 4, 5, 56–58
Pyridoxine, 66, 70
Pyrrolizidine, 110

Quick freezing, 19
Quillaia, 25

R groups, 57, 58
RDA (recommended daily allowances),
  71
Rennet, 59
Rennin, 59
Reproductive defects, 100
Research, 10
Riboflavin, 65, 70
Rice, 3
Rickets, 4

Saccharin, 54, 56, 78
Saccharomuces spp., 60
Safety margins, 7
Safety testing, xiv, 27, 94–105
Safrole, 107, 108
Salmonella, 100
Salt, 11, 12
Saponin, 25
Saturated compound, 14
Saxitoxin, 114
Screening tests, 96, 100

126